FOOT CARE BOOK

Runner's World

FOOT CARE BOOK

by Dennis R. Zamzow, D.P.M.
& William P. Feigel, D.P.M.

Runner's World Books

Library of Congress Cataloging in Publication Data

Zamzow, Dennis; Feigel, William
    Foot care book.

    (Instructional book series;# 15)
    1. Foot — Care and hygiene.
    I. Feigel, William.
II. Title.
RD563.Z25   1982   617' .585   82-21625
ISBN 0-89037-233-0   (spiral)
ISBN 0-89037-245-4   (pbk.)

Illustrated by Mary Shyne and Kevin J. Moran

Runner's World Books
in conjunction with
Anderson World, Inc., Mountain View, CA

Contents

Introduction I

When I was asked to co-author a book about foot and leg care I was initially flattered. This feeling soon passed to be replaced by fear, then terror. How was I going to fill an entire book about foot-related problems? I soon learned, as I guess every first-time author does, that sparsity gives way to abundance. After I started researching and writing, I realized that the problem was not one of coming up with enough information, but of paring away the reams of information I had gathered.

I hope this book is clear, concise and simple enough to understand. I have talked with numerous non-medical people who have read similar books. To a person they complained that these books are too technical. I hope this problem has been eliminated here — not by talking down to the reader but by presenting the information clearly and in appropriate order.

The fitness boom that has made us healthy has also increased the number of overuse injuries we see in the office. Many of these injuries can be avoided with common sense and an understanding of why injuries occur. This, in essence, is the content of our book.

There is not enough room to mention all the people who have made this book possible. I do want to give special thanks to *Runner's World* for giving the opportunity to write a book. A special thanks goes to my partner Dennis Zamzow, who is an inspiration to work with.

Two other people played an integral part in assembling this book. Heidi Ness spent many hours typing the manuscript while carrying out her office duties and attending school. Cindy Zamarrow managed to put up with me the many months I spent writing. Without her inspiration, occasional prodding, typing, dictation and editing skills this book would not be in front of you.

Finally, I thank the patients who had enough confidence in me to let me treat them. Experience is the great teacher. Together, we still have much to learn.

William Feigel, D.P.M.
Mountain View, California
September 1982

Introduction II

When I began this introduction my mind filled with the names of everyone who made this book possible, but then the book would be filled with names spanning a lifetime. And in essence, that's what the book is about, a lifetime of learning and experience put into words. From following my dad behind the tractor in Wisconsin at age four to running a one hundred-mile endurance run at age thirty-eight. To everyone I met in between — I thank you.

And special thanks go to a few other people: *Runner's World* for making this book possible; Heidi Ness for staying until 11 p.m. typing many a night; and my partner Bill Feigel.

This book is for you, the reader. I hope by the knowledge you gain here your run will be more pleasant or your activity becomes injury-free. So much of this book is from first-hand experience — the fifth metatarsal fracture from stepping on an unexposed root to the blisters in a marathon; the muscle pull from that extra effort in the quarter-mile to the tendinitis from soft shoes after the first six-miler; the unbelievable joy of finishing the first marathon to the splendor of the trails in a sunlit woods. I hope all this comes through in the book.

And finally, special thanks to you Mom and Dad, for without you, this book would not have been.

Dennis R. Zamzow, D.P.M.
Mountain View, California
September 1982

1

The Structure of the Foot

The logical way to write a book about the human foot is to start by explaining the parts that make up the structure. The human foot is extremely complex — its elegantly designed parts sophisticated and well integrated. There is much more to the foot than just five toes and some bones covered by skin.

Understanding the foot's functions and injuries requires a basic knowledge of its physiology. As an analogy, think of the apprentice car mechanic who must first learn the individual parts of the engine before he can comprehend their function. He is taught the conceptual relationships of the parts as they work together. Only after he understands these parts and their interactions can he be a full-fledged mechanic. So it is with the human body. You must identify and study parts of the human anatomy to understand how the body functions.

Mention the word anatomy and many think they're going to get lost in medical school lingo. While anatomy can be a difficult subject, in this book we will present the topic from a point of view that will make it easy to understand; you will get a better idea of what lies under the skin. As you read what follows, keep in mind one idea — you are living in your own lab. Every structure we describe is contained in your foot and leg. If, for example, we talk about knee function, roll up a pant leg and watch your knee flex. This practice will make easier the understanding of the structure and function of the parts. By understanding your foot, ankle and leg you can understand how injuries in these areas occur, how to treat them and, more importantly, how to prevent them.

For a moment, think of yourself as a manufacturer with unlimited resources and talent. Your latest assignment is to construct a foot and leg. You've been given the plans and all the parts you need to work with; all you have to do is put them together on your assembly line. Here we will proceed to build a foot, and then a leg.

BONES

Any structure — whether it be a car, house or even a bird cage — must start with a framework. It is upon this lattice or framework that a product will be produced. The framework must on the one hand be strong enough to withstand the forces that act upon the final product and at the same time be small enough so as not to overwhelm the final structure.

Bone is an ideal frame material around which to build the body. Bone is light, yet can endure tremendous stress, and it can repair itself.

The foot is made of twenty-eight individual, identifiable bones. Fig. 1-1a, b shows the bones of the foot and their names. Note the complexity of the bone structure of the foot; now note their positions as you look at your own feet. It's not important that you remember individual bones, but be aware of the different sections — toes, forefoot and rearfoot, which are shown in the diagram. Also note the sesamoid bones. These two pea-shaped bones under the ball of the foot at the first metatarsal are often injured; you'll read more about injury to these bones in future chapters.

An X-ray from the top and side of the human foot is shown in Fig. 1-2a, b. X-rays depict nicely a three-dimensional object on a two-dimensional plate; they are an important and vital tool to the podiatrist diagnosing an injury. We are showing you this X-ray of a "normal" foot so that you may refer back to it when we present X-rays of abnormalities or injuries to the foot in upcoming chapters. Remember that X-rays only show solid objects, like bones, so none of the other soft tissue structures that surround bones will appear — ligaments, tendons, muscles, nerves, blood vessels, etc. Now, let's find out how these twenty-eight bones are held together.

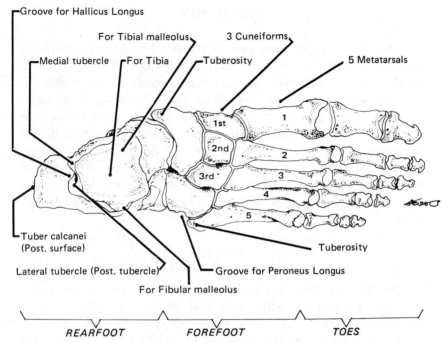

Groove for Hallicus Longus

For Tibial malleolus

3 Cuneiforms

5 Metatarsals

Medial tubercle

For Tibia

Tuberosity

1st

2nd

3rd

1

2

3

4

5

Tuber calcanei
(Post. surface)

Lateral tubercle (Post. tubercle)

For Fibular malleolus

Groove for Peroneus Longus

Tuberosity

REARFOOT

FOREFOOT

TOES

Fig. 1-1a   The Bones of the Foot (dorsal aspect)

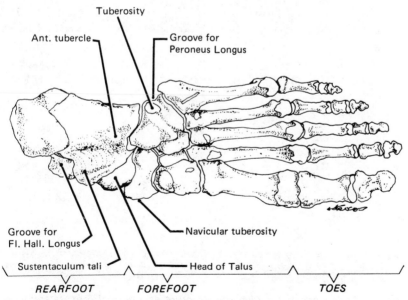

Tuberosity

Ant. tubercle

Groove for
Peroneus Longus

Groove for
Fl. Hall. Longus

Navicular tuberosity

Sustentaculum tali

Head of Talus

REARFOOT

FOREFOOT

TOES

Fig. 1-1b   The Bones of the Foot (plantar aspect)   (after Clement's)

LIGAMENTS

Nature has created ligaments to act as a biological glue to hold bones and other structures together. Ligaments are made of a tough, fibrous material that has the consistency of gristle. In Fig. 1-3 you can see that several of these ligaments hold bones together. There are over two hundred individual, identifiable, ligaments in the foot — each with a specific role of holding tightly the bones it attaches to. Remember that ligaments are strongest at their attachment points and weakest at the area farthest from attachment points, or the "center." This is important when considering ligament injuries, which will be discussed throughout the book.

JOINTS

Now that we have attached all the ligaments to the bones, the foot is taking shape. Now, note that where the bones connect, they grate against each other when moved. This is the joint. A joint is a point where two bones come together. Joints are particularly important in the foot since there are many bones (such as the toes) that move at every step you take.

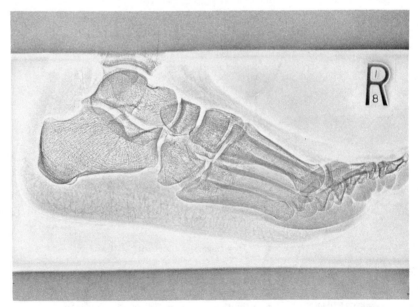

Fig. 1-2a *Xerogram showing the structure of a normal foot (lateral view).*

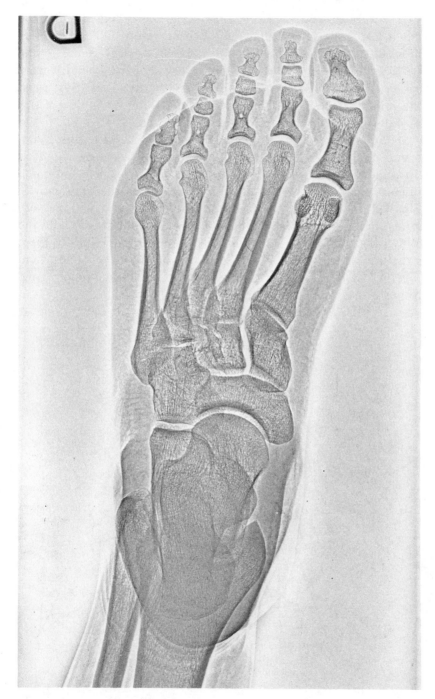

Fig. 1-2b *Xerogram showing the structure of a normal foot (dorsal view).*

If raw bone were to rub on raw bone, soon there wouldn't be much left — to say nothing of the pain you would endure. But then there's cartilage, which covers bone surfaces at the joints. Cartilage is white, it glistens, and is very slippery — as if it were covered with oil. Perfect, you think, as you attach cartilage to all the joint surfaces. But then you wonder, how do I protect this obviously delicate cartilage?; back to the plans.

In order to protect the joints and at the same time supply nutrients and lubricating fluid to the joint surfaces, each joint is surrounded by a capsule. This capsule is like a ligament but much thicker, and is pliable to allow for bending as the joint moves. Fig. 1-4 shows a typical joint capsule. Integrated within every joint capsule are several ligaments whose function it is to hold the joint stable and at the same time allow for motion. Injury to these structures is quite common. So now you have the bones, held together by the ligaments and the joints, protected and functioning. Now the muscles.

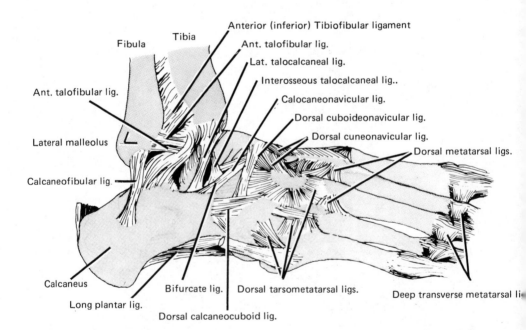

Fig. 1-3 Ligaments of the Foot

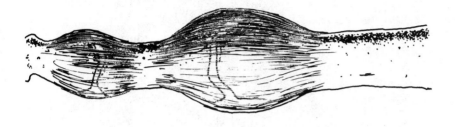

Fig. 1-4 Joint Capsule

MUSCLES

Muscles are what allow joints to move. Muscles are the work-horse of the body. They provide the mechanical energy of motion and, indeed, of life — remember the heart is a large muscle. In the foot there are more than twenty muscles, which are shown in Fig. 1-5a-e. Note that there is only one muscle on the top of the foot; the rest are layered on the bottom (bottom in anatomical parlance is known as plantar) of the foot.

But how does the muscle manage to pull on a particular bone to allow for motion? This function is performed through the tendons. Tendons and muscles must be thought of as a continuum. For instance, Fig. 1-6 shows the calf muscles and the Achilles tendon. Notice that the muscle mass is high up on the leg, but as the muscle courses down the leg it gradually forms the Achilles tendon, which attaches to the heel bone. When the muscle works, the tendon is pulled and the heel bone, to which the tendon is attached, moves. As an analogy, think of the muscle as a winch that has power. The rope is attached to the winch and the rope itself is

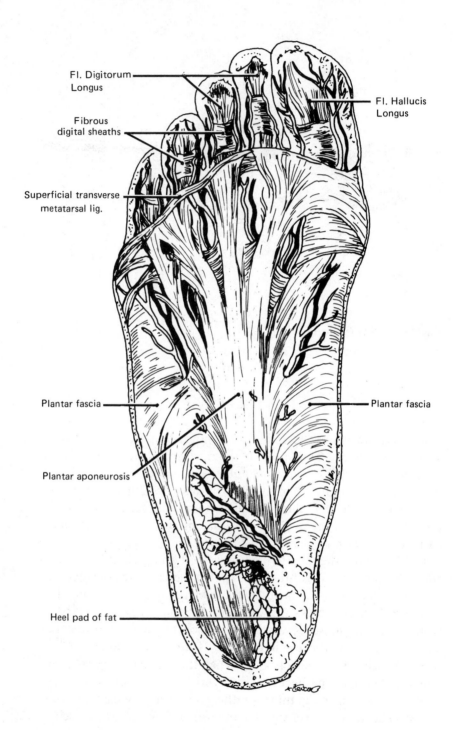

Fl. Digitorum Longus

Fibrous digital sheaths

Superficial transverse metatarsal lig.

Fl. Hallucis Longus

Plantar fascia

Plantar fascia

Plantar aponeurosis

Heel pad of fat

Fig. 1-5a Superficial dissection of foot (plantar view)

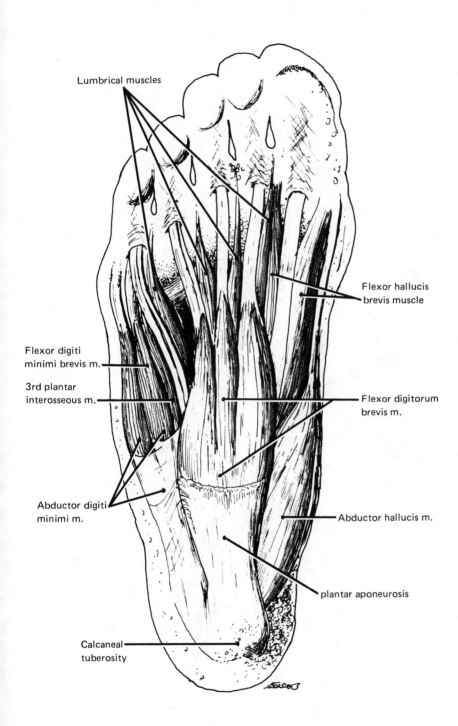

Lumbrical muscles

Flexor hallucis
brevis muscle

Flexor digiti
minimi brevis m.

3rd plantar
interosseous m.

Flexor digitorum
brevis m.

Abductor digiti
minimi m.

Abductor hallucis m.

plantar aponeurosis

Calcaneal
tuberosity

Fig. 1-5b   The first layer of plantar muscles

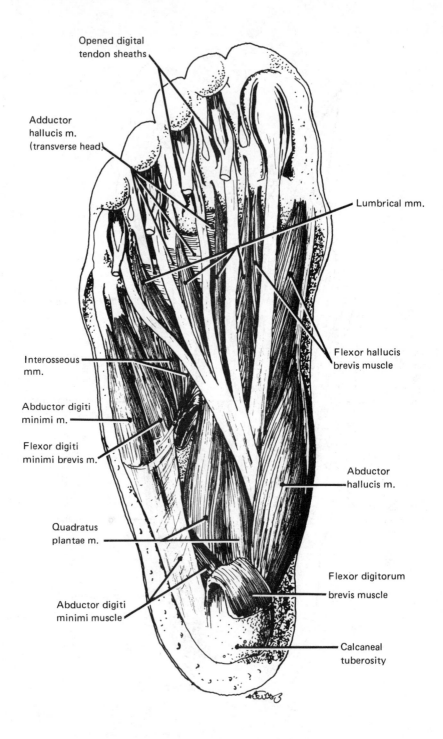

Opened digital
tendon sheaths

Adductor
hallucis m.
(transverse head)

Lumbrical mm.

Flexor hallucis
brevis muscle

Interosseous
mm.

Abductor digiti
minimi m.

Flexor digiti
minimi brevis m.

Abductor
hallucis m.

Quadratus
plantae m.

Flexor digitorum
brevis muscle

Abductor digiti
minimi muscle

Calcaneal
tuberosity

Fig. 1-5c   The second layer of plantar muscles

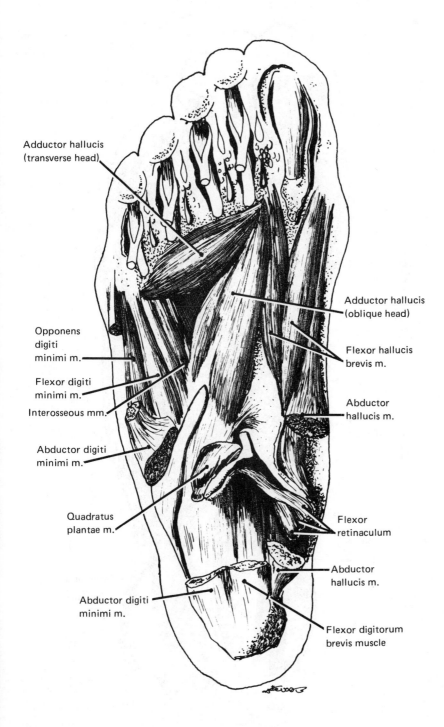

Adductor hallucis
(transverse head)

Opponens
digiti
minimi m.

Flexor digiti
minimi m.

Interosseous mm.

Abductor digiti
minimi m.

Quadratus
plantae m.

Abductor digiti
minimi m.

Adductor hallucis
(oblique head)

Flexor hallucis
brevis m.

Abductor
hallucis m.

Flexor
retinaculum

Abductor
hallucis m.

Flexor digitorum
brevis muscle

Fig. 1-5d   The third layer of plantar muscles

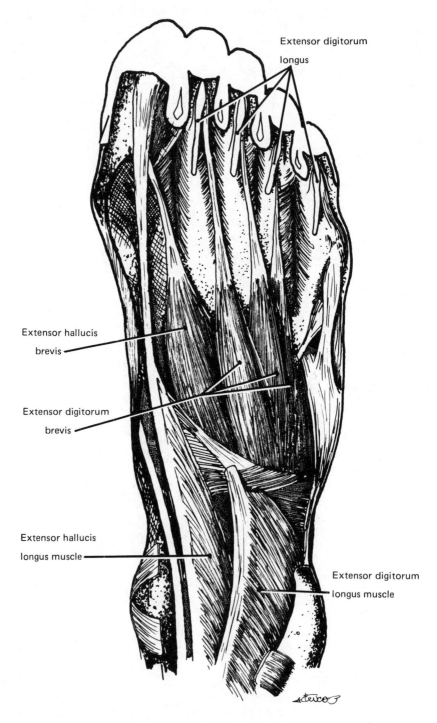

Extensor digitorum longus

Extensor hallucis brevis

Extensor digitorum brevis

Extensor hallucis longus muscle

Extensor digitorum longus muscle

Fig. 1-5e The muscles of the foot (dorsal view)

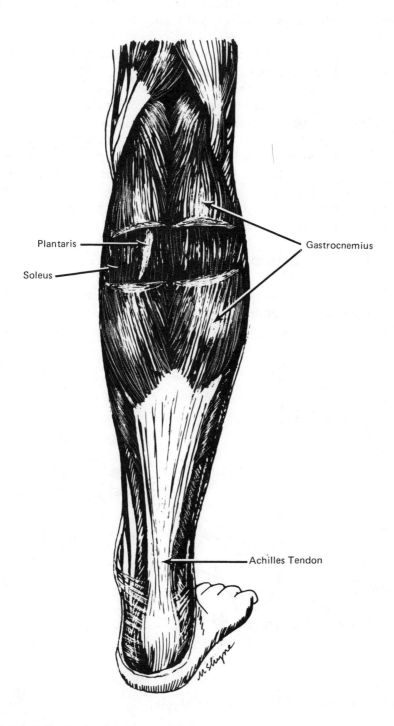

Plantaris

Soleus

Gastrocnemius

Achilles Tendon

Fig. 1-6 Posterior Lower Leg Muscles

attached to the object to be moved. When the winch (muscle) is activated, the rope (tendon) pulls taught and the load (bone) moves.

Fig. 1-7 shows a typical joint with its associated tendons. Here we have shown the first metatarsal-phalangeal joint — the big toe joint. When the flexor tendon (on the bottom) or extensor tendon moves, the joint will move down or up, respectively.

There are two types of muscle fibers — slow twitch and fast twitch. Each of us is born with a certain percentage of slow-twitch and fast-twitch fibers. Slow-twitch muscle fibers have greater endurance than fast twitch. On the other hand, the fast-twitch fibers allow for quick acceleration, and they deplete themselves of energy quickly. A marathon runner uses mostly the slow-twitch fibers, while a sprinter employs fast-twitch fibers.

BLOOD VESSELS AND NERVES

Now that the bones, ligaments and muscles are in place, we must provide nourishment and sensory information to the foot. These functions are carried out by the blood vessels and nerves,

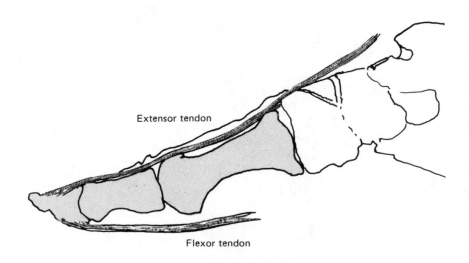

Extensor tendon

Flexor tendon

Fig. 1-7 First metatarsal-phalangeal joint

respectively. The foot is well supplied with nerves; this is so that you can better perceive the position of your foot on the ground.

Conversely, the blood supply to the foot, as opposed to the rest of the body, is poor. The reason is twofold. First, the foot is the farthest structure from the heart and, second, in normal ambulation the effects of gravity tend to work against adequate blood flow. This fact is important when one considers vascular problems in the foot and leg, which will be discussed in detail in subsequent chapters.

Well, at this point the bones, ligaments, muscles, tendons, nerves and blood vessels all fit together nicely. All we need now is some skin.

SKIN

Skin is an organ (excretory and absorptive), which makes it the largest in the body. It must protect the anatomy underneath it and yet allow fluids in and out. It must be tough to withstand the lumps, bumps and bruises of daily activity and yet be pliable to allow for bending at each motion of the body. In addition, skin must protect itself from the deleterious effects of ultraviolet light and other damaging environmental factors by rapidly repairing itself. Skin must be able to, in every square millimeter, distinguish hot from cold, wet from dry, and have great sensitivity. The skin on your feet must be tough enough to withstand constant pounding, yet remain sensitive to the elements.

The skin has two major layers, known as the dermis and epidermis. The dermis is the deep layer that contains growing cells. As these cells mature they are pushed to the surface and eventually die, forming the epidermis, or dead outer layer. The dermal layer also contains skin pigment cells, blood vessels, nerves and hair follicles that make up the skin.

The bottom of the foot, because of the increased pressure demands, has developed a mechanism whereby the epidermal layer grows much thicker than elsewhere on the body. This extra protection cushions the bottom of the foot; however, the thickened epidermal layer is more prone to injury on the bottom of the foot. Thicker skin also has a greater tendency to become dry. Dry skin tends to crack, which invites infection and abrasions. Skin problems will be discussed in Chapter 5.

LEG

The leg has three bones — the femur, the tibia and the fibula. The femur is the thigh bone, and the tibia and fibula make up the lower leg. The two bones connect at the knee joint, as shown in Fig. 1-8. The lower end of the tibia and fibula articulate (form a joint) with the foot at the ankle joint. The ankle joint is shown in Fig. 1-9. It is the muscles of the lower leg that have the most profound effect on foot function. There are ten important muscles in the lower leg originating at the tibia and fibula and that send tendons to attach at the foot. These are known as the extrinsic muscles since they originate from outside of the foot. Because these muscles have a major influence on foot function they are very susceptible to injury.

Refer to Figs. 1-6 and 1-12. The calf muscle has three components. The outermost muscles, as shown, are known as the gastrocnemius. These originate from above the knee joint; the importance of this will be shown later. The "gastrocs" extend to form the Achilles tendon, which attaches to the heel bone. Beneath the gastrocs is a large muscle attached to the tibia and fibula.

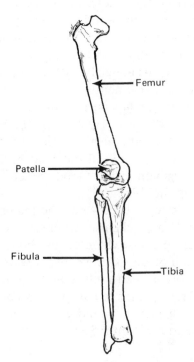

Femur

Patella

Fibula

Tibia

Fig. 1-8   Bones of the Leg

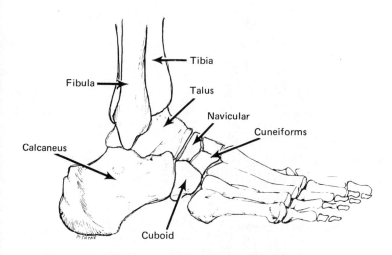

Fig. 1-9 Attachment of the Leg to the Ankle

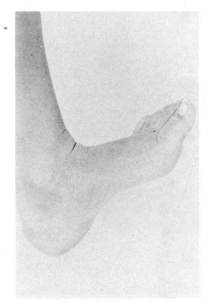

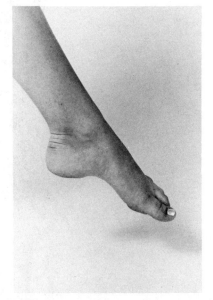

Fig. 1-10a Dorsiflexion.   **Fig. 1-10b Plantarflexion.**

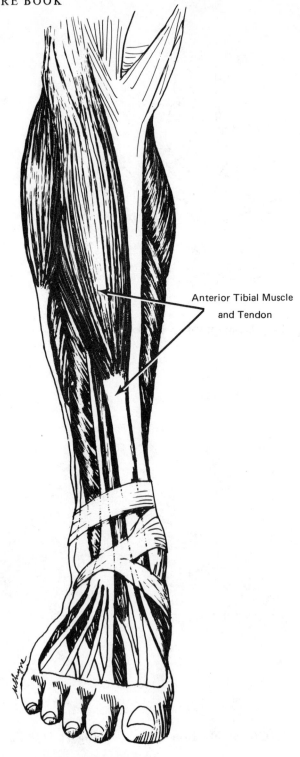

Anterior Tibial Muscle
and Tendon

Fig. 1-11   Anterior Lower Leg Muscles

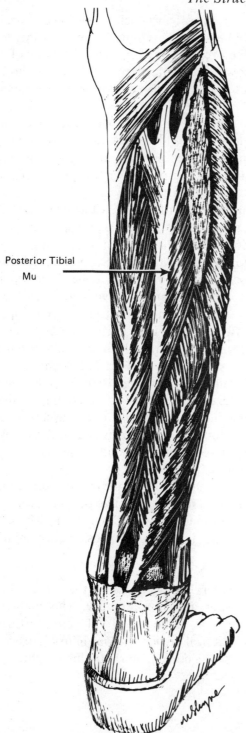

Posterior Tibial
Mu

Fig. 1-12   Posterior Lower Leg Muscles (Deeper Layer)

Called the soleus muscle, its origin is below the knee — again an important point to remember. This muscle, in addition to the gastrocs, makes up the Achilles tendon. The function of these muscles is to pull down or plantarflex the foot, as shown in Fig. 1-10. The gastrocs/soleus muscles also allow you to stand on your toes.

On the front of the leg is the anterior tibial muscle and tendon. This muscle, as shown in Fig. 1-11, is responsible for pulling the foot up, or dorsiflexing it. Moreover, this muscle is usually related with that common, nagging injury known as shinsplints. Read Chapter 8 for more on shinsplints.

On the medial (inside) portion of the leg, attached to the tibia, is the posterior tibial muscle. This is a deep leg muscle, as shown in Fig. 1-12. The posterior tibial pulls the foot as shown in Fig. 3-5. — a motion that is known as inversion or supination. Posterior tibial tendinitis is also a common injury, to be discussed later.

The final muscles to consider are the two known as the peroneals. These muscles originate on the outside of the upper leg and course down the fibula. Their tendons pass behind the ankle joint. The peroneal brevis (shorter muscle) attaches to the base of the fifth metatarsal, as shown in Fig. 6-2. The point of attachment is an important consideration when discussing ankle injuries. The peroneus longus courses under the foot, attaching to the ball of the foot at the first metatarsal. These two muscles have the function of pulling the foot out, as shown in Fig. 3-1. This motion is known as eversion, or pronation, and these muscles act as antagonists to the posterior tibial muscles.

The muscles we have discussed play a role in foot function. The muscles are vulnerable to injury in the active person because they play an active role in movement. By understanding where these muscles are and how they function, diagnosing foot injuries is made easier.

In the following chapters we will discuss the more common injuries we see in our sportsmedicine practice. This book is not just a self-treatment manual, although it will help you identify your injury and offer practical advice. If your injury persists after rest and self-treatment, professional help should be sought.

2

The Foot and Leg in Motion

Now that we have the foot and leg assembled, they attach to the body at the hip. The hip joint, as does the shoulder joint, has three directions of motion. Unlike the knee, which only moves up and down, the hip can move in any direction. Such joint mobility is often implicated with injuries, which will be discussed in Chapter 10.

The foot contacts the ground first; it takes the majority of stress generated at each step. Dr. Roger Mann has quantified the amount of stress an individual's foot experiences while running. According to Dr. Mann, "Considering that there are about eight hundred footstrikes by each foot in a one-mile run, and given a one hundred fifty-pound person running this distance, each foot must endure about one hundred twenty tons of force. In a marathon, (26.2 miles) each foot must endure three thousand tons of force." Needless to say, it is crucial that the foot function properly in order to accommodate this stress. By understanding the mechanisms of force dissipation in the foot, you can better comprehend injuries and recognize a potential problem before damage is done.

NORMAL FOOT FUNCTION

Throughout this chapter and in subsequent chapters some key terms will be introduced. Be sure their meanings are clear, or you may have difficulty understanding how an injury occurs.

The most important joint when considering foot function is the subtalar joint. This joint is directly below the ankle joint, as shown in Fig. 2-1. It has a complex set of motions that, when functioning normally, allow the foot to dissipate the majority of force generated at each step. This joint's vital role is illustrated in Fig. 2-2a — a rear view of the right foot and leg at heel contact during the gait cycle. The heel's position reflects that of the subtalar joint (for simplicity, we can interchange the terms subtalar joint and heel). Note that the forefoot is not yet on the ground and that the heel contacts the ground on the outside of the foot. The first part of the foot to make ground contact, then, is the outside of the heel. This heel-turned-in position is known as *inversion* or *supination.*

The footplant cycle continues in Fig. 2-2b, where the forefoot comes closer to being flat on the ground. The heel now assumes a perpendicular position under the leg. This is known as the heel's *neutral position.*

As the forefoot contacts the ground and begins to bear weight, the heel turns out in relation to the lower leg. This position (shown in Fig. 2-2c) is known as *eversion* or *pronation.*

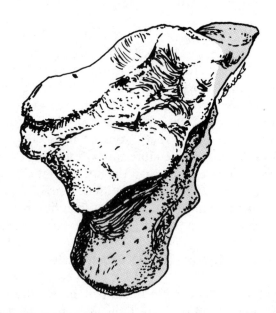

Fig. 2-1 Subtalar Joint *(highlighted area accommodates talar)*

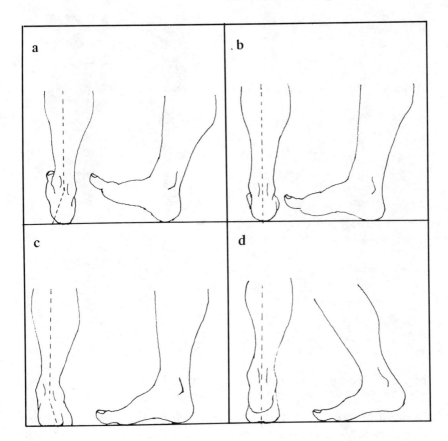

Fig. 2-2 The Gait Cycle

As the cycle continues, the heel begins to lift off the ground. The heel reverses its direction and returns to its *neutral position* (Fig. 2-2d), and then to a position of *supination*.

This movement of the heel is essential for proper foot function. A person's impact, in terms of body weight, increases three- to four-fold when the foot contacts the ground while running. This force, to be rendered harmless, must be controlled and dissipated evenly. If it is not controlled, injury can occur in the foot, ankle, knee, hip or lower back.

The precise mechanism within the subtalar joint is complex and will not be discussed at this time. Basically, the foot, in order to dissipate these forces, must follow the motions outlined here — from supination at heel contact to neutral position, to pronation and back to supination at toe-off. Any alteration can lead to injury.

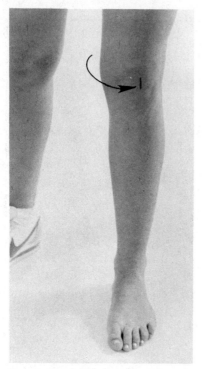 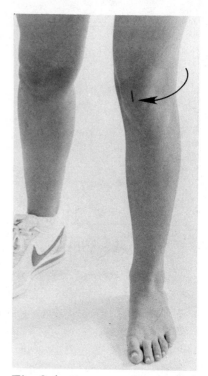

Fig. 2-3 *The supinated foot causes the knee to rotate outward.*

Fig. 2-4 *The pronated foot causes the knee to rotate inward.*

In addition to the subtalar joint dissipating force, consider this: For a variety of complex reasons, when the foot is supinated it becomes rigid. In other words, it behaves as a single unit or what has come to be known as a rigid lever. Conversely, when the foot pronates it becomes very loose or, as has been termed, the foot becomes a bag of bones. The implications are important at each step. At heel contact the foot is rigid and quickly pronates as the foot bears weight, and then becomes very loose, for good reason: A loose bag of bones will adapt much better to an uneven surface compared to a rigid foot. In other words, a pronated foot can adapt to rough terrain — an inherited, evolutionary trait. By the same token, as the foot propels itself forward at toe-off it should be supinated. Remember that a supinated foot is rigid, which is ideal for propulsion.

The mechanism of force dissipation, propulsion and adaptation as the foot moves from a supinated to a pronated and supinated position at each step is a complex one; it is essential for normal foot and leg function. Any alteration to the forces or structures that contribute to this mechanism can lead to injury.

THE LEG IN NORMAL MOTION

When the foot moves so does everything else it is connected to — the ankle, knee, hip, leg and pelvis. To put it simply — everything relates. Every action of one part of the body has an effect on all the other structures that surround it.

As you will recall, the normal foot moves from a position of supination at heel contact to pronation until forefoot contact and back to supination at toe-off. This motion also forces the leg to move from external rotation to internal rotation at every step. Or, consider the kneecap as an indicator of the position of the leg. When the foot is in its neutral position the kneecap (and hence the leg) is pointed straight ahead. If the foot is supinated, the kneecap now points out, as shown in Fig. 2-3. This is known as external rotation of the leg. Conversely, when the foot is pronated the kneecap (leg) turns in, as shown in Fig. 2-4. This is known as internal rotation. You may wonder what all this means. Well, if the foot is overly pronated or supinated, the leg will spend too much time in an internal or external rotated position. Thus, all the structures (muscles, joints, bones) of the leg are stressed; the stage is set for injury.

In addition to the foot causing excessive internal or external rotation of the leg, an abnormally functioning foot can affect the position of the pelvis, which in turn leads to undue stress on the back; it can also cause sciatica. More on this later.

The foot has a direct and profound effect on the leg and back; we cannot emphasize this enough. These concepts in this chapter and the accompanying terminology are crucial to your understanding the next chapters. Terminology here appears over and over again in upcoming chapters.

3

Abnormal Foot Function

If the "ideal" situation — the foot and leg in perfect alignment as described — were normal, there would be no need for this book. But reality rarely recognizes the ideal. In fact, a recent survey has shown that more than 90 percent of all people have some type of biomechanical imbalance within the foot. These abnormalities are dealt with in biomechanics — the study of the body in motion.

Biomechanics attempts to relate normal to abnormal body function. In other words, by knowing how a normal foot and leg functions you can better understand how abnormal forces can lead to overuse and injury. The abnormality that causes the most problems for the active person is overpronation.

OVERPRONATION

The foot should strike the ground in a supinated position at heelstrike. This is followed by immediate pronation as the foot bears weight and the forefoot contacts the ground. Resupination follows as the heel lifts off the ground. With overpronation, the foot remains in the pronated position throughout the gait cycle. Supination does not occur, therefore the forces that normally would be eliminated by the foot are allowed to extend up the leg. The stage is now set for injuries such as ankle sprains, heel spurs, shinsplints, knee pain, hip and back pain, etc.

For example, look at the individual in Fig. 3-1 — a runner with overpronated feet. In Fig. 3-2, the same individual has his feet placed in their neutral position. Note that the heel is directly under the leg. This is the position that this individual's foot should be in for normal function.

There are several ways to self-diagnose overpronation. First, have someone watch you walk. If you are overpronating, your foot will tend to roll in. Second, examine your sports shoes. These are probably the best indicator of a foot problem. If the foot is functioning normally, the bottoms of the shoes should wear as shown in Fig. 3-3 — on the outside of the heel and the inside of the ball of the foot. But more important, place the shoes on a table and examine the position of the heel. If the foot functions normally, the heel will be perpendicular to the surface, as you would find in a new shoe. If, however, the foot overpronates, the shoe will begin to wear according to how the heel (and, hence, the foot) functions. In Fig. 3-4 we show two-month-old running shoes from an individual who overpronates severely. Note that the bisection of the heel is skewed in the direction of overpronation.

So you might say, "Big deal if my foot overpronates. I don't have any problems with injuries." Fine. However, this analogy might make you think twice: A car is slightly out of tune. The car gets you where you want to go, but it's not running as efficiently or as smoothly as it could. The potential for damage to that car's engine is greater than with the tuned engine. So it is with a foot that is "slightly out of tune." If you do suffer from nagging injuries to the foot, ankle, knee, hip, or even back, then consider the foot as the source of the problem. In the words of Dr. George Sheehan, when discussing how to treat runner's knee, "You treat the foot."

There are other long-term problems that stem from overpronation. Contrary to popular belief, you do not get a flat foot (a simplistic term for overpronation) from wearing inferior shoes as a child. Overpronation is determined solely (pardon the pun) by genetics. At birth, the shape your foot will grow to is predetermined. Shoes have little to do with changing the shape of your foot. They frequently aggravate a problem that is already present, however. Secondary problems such as bunions, heel spurs, plantar fasciitis and hammer toes are caused by overpronation.

Overpronation is corrected by reducing the excessive movement of the foot during pronation. Better shoes are often recommended. In more severe cases, a commercial or homemade felt wedge, with the high part on the inside, can be placed in the heel of the shoe so

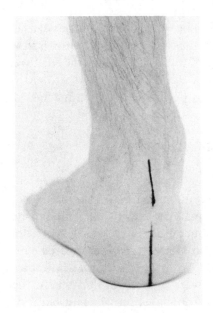

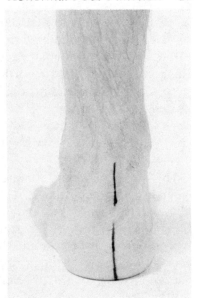

Fig. 3-1 *Overpronated.*

Fig. 3-2 *Neutral.*

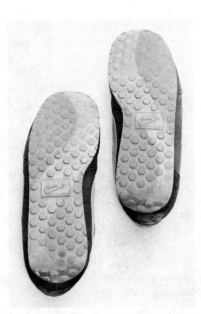

Fig. 3-3 *Highlighted area shows serpentine pattern of normal shoe wear.*

as to slightly supinate the foot. If you suffer from injuries caused by overpronation, the best treatment is to use an orthotic, a shoe insert that will place your foot back in its proper neutral position. Chapter 10 is devoted to orthotics. No matter what treatment is necessary, the important point is to determine why injury has occurred.

OVERSUPINATION

This problem is less common than overpronation, but afflicts enough active people that it deserves mention. As the name implies, oversupination occurs when the foot spends too much of its time as shown in Fig. 3-5. Remember that the foot, at heel contact, should strike the ground in a supinated position. When a foot oversupinates, its restricted range of motion does not allow pronation. In other words, because the foot turns out so much, the foot can't pronate adequately; the foot jams into its end range of motion and can move no farther. Unlike the foot that pronates excessively and is flexible, the oversupinated foot is rigid. The resulting lack of shock absorption leads to injury.

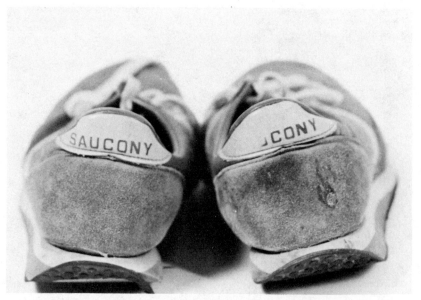

Fig. 3-4 *The two-month-old running shoes of an individual who overpronates severely.*

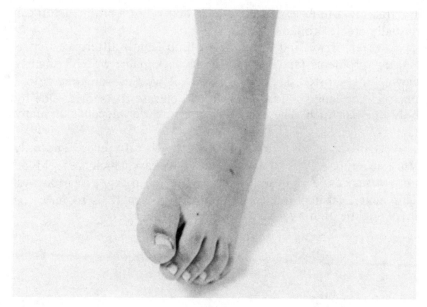

Fig. 3-5 *The foot in a supinated position.*

An oversupinated foot is one that has a very high arch. Treatment is aimed at supplying the foot with some type of shock absorber. This can be done in a number of ways: First, use shoes with softer soles. Second, use a cushion insert. Insoles, such as Spenco, are good for shock absorption. Third, pursue your activity on a softer surface. For instance, if you are a runner, train on grass, on trails or on a track. Ideally, the best treatment is a semi-rigid orthotic that functions as a shock absorber while also controlling foot function.

LIMB LENGTH DIFFERENCE

Surprisingly, more than 75 percent of the population has some degree of limb length difference. However, the vast majority of these individuals have no symptoms related to this problem. The body adapts to the difference in a variety of ways. The pelvis will tilt, the foot attached to the longer leg will overpronate, thereby making the leg functionally shorter, or else the spine will tilt. No matter what the method, the body adapts itself to the difference in leg length. In this example, if we discover someone with a limb length difference and it is not symptomatic, then we leave it alone.

By treating a limb length difference that is not a problem you can actually create problems.

However, if we find a significant limb length difference that is causing problems (such as low-grade back pain) we will slightly elevate the shorter side. For instance, if we find someone with a one-inch leg length difference, we will elevate the shorter side by only one-half inch. The exact amount, however, depends on many factors.

It is difficult to measure a limb length difference. The only truly accurate way is to do a full-body X-ray, which we feel is an unnecessary expense in addition to an unneeded exposure to X-rays. The next best method to determine limb length is to have the individual lie on his back and to measure the legs.

4

The Reason for Injury

Injuries, obviously, vary as to severity. Most activity-related injuries are often caused by overuse. In this chapter we are not discussing injuries that occur, for instance, when you are run over by a Mack truck, or broadsided by a two hundred fifty-pound linebacker. Obviously these injuries are caused by direct trauma, and not overuse.

As stated, overuse is the major cause of injury athletes are most familiar with. Overuse is defined as abnormal stress placed on any structure within the body. This undue stress causes microtrauma to a given structure, and can be thought of as putting stress on an area such that it is unable to cope. Common overuse injuries we see include runner's knee, shinsplints, stress fractures, heel spurs, tendinitis and muscle strains.

The purpose of training, or for that matter doing any type of exercise, is to effect a beneficial change to your body. This encompasses improving muscular development, increasing the aerobic/cardiovascular threshold, preventing heart disease, or just looking trim and feeling healthy.

The key to taking up any type of exercise is gradual adaptation. For example, when you start running don't expect to be able to run ten miles the first workout. Your body must first develop stronger muscles in the leg and foot and increase cardiovascular capability for endurance.

Training is the process of overtaxing the body and then building it back up so that it is stronger than it was at the outset. But this must be done gradually and using common sense. Back to your running. If you can run comfortably at ten miles a week, then the next step would be to increase your mileage. However, increase it by only 10 to 15 percent every two weeks. The body can then strengthen gradually with less chance of injury. If too much stress is placed on the body by overexercising, then the stage is set for injury. If you're lucky, no injury will occur and the body will strengthen. But if microtrauma occurs, the physiological response is inflammation.

INFLAMMATION

Any time muscles, tendons or ligaments are overstressed, pulled, torn or injured, the body immediately reacts to repair the injury. First, there is an immediate constriction or narrowing of the blood vessels in the injured area. This prevents significant blood loss at the outset of the injury. Almost immediately after constriction begins there is a dilation, or opening, of the blood vessels. For example, when you are pricked by a pin, the puncture doesn't bleed for a couple of seconds, but then it begins to bleed profusely.

Once the blood vessels dilate, fluid from the blood is exuded into the injured area. This is not blood; rather, it is body fluid containing various cells and material that will begin the repair process. If the injury is severe, blood vessels will rupture and blood will leak out under the skin, which will show as a black-and-blue mark. However, in most overuse injuries blood vessels are not broken, hence there is no noticeable bruising.

After several minutes fluid will have accumulated around the injured area, and there will be swelling. This swelling is a normal physiological response of the body as it attempts to repair the injury. Remember that within this fluid are the cells and materials necessary for the repair process to take place. Over time, several hours to days, the cells within this fluid in and around the injured area become very active and proliferate as the repair proceeds. These cells produce collagen, which acts like a glue and helps hold the body together. This entire process of repair is known as inflammation.

Concern yourself with controlling the inflammatory process. This is not to imply that you should stop the inflammation;

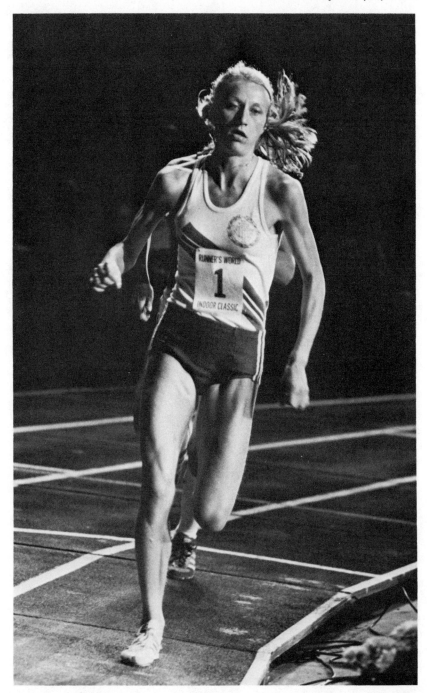

Fig. 4-1 *Grete Waitz avoids injury through proper training.*

rather, the treatment should be aimed at reducing the inflammation to a tolerable pain level and combating swelling.

Ice is the recommended treatment when an injury first occurs. Ice cools the tissues and thus constricts the surrounding blood vessels that are attempting to dilate and exude fluid. Because less fluid is delivered to the injured area, swelling is lessened.

The old saying, "An ounce of prevention is worth a pound of cure," is true for the active individual. The basic rule for all athletes to avoid minor injury is to follow gradual adaptation.

We will discuss the various treatments of injuries in the upcoming chapters. But once an injury occurs you should stop all activity, get treatment, and find out why the injury occurred. We have seen many active people in our offices who have been injured, and treated their injuries lightly. By not finding out why they got injured, their problems only worsened.

5

Forefoot Problems

TOENAILS

Primitive man used his toenails for climbing, digging or fighting. They were often broken or otherwise injured. Today, the runner — with all the various types of shoes and terrain that he encounters — faces many of the same problems. We will discuss the most common ailments you may experience and how to deal with them.

Probably the most frequent toenail problem we see is the traumatically avulsed toenail, whereby the nail is partially torn from its bed. Fortunately, endorphins (morphine-like, naturally occurring chemicals) that are generated during activity mask the pain. After you stop the activity, however, and the shoe and sock are taken off, you may experience pain and notice bleeding. Sometimes the nail is completely pulled off the toe, or more likely there will be just minor hemorrhaging beneath the nail, causing a small black-and-blue mark. If there is continual bleeding and the nail is totally avulsed (a tearing away forcefully of the whole nail) or even partially avulsed and hanging, seek professional help. If there is just a small black-and-blue mark but you have considerable pain, here's what to do: Heat a paper clip with a match; then use the tip of the paper clip to melt through the top of the nail into the area where there is accumulated blood. Blood will probably then spurt or ooze out of the hole, and the pain will be relieved. This easy procedure does not hurt, but if you are a little squeamish, have a friend do it. After relieving the pressure, apply a topical antibiotic and a Band-Aid or small dressing over the nail.

If a considerable portion of the nail is torn away from the nail bed and a good portion underneath the nail is black-and-blue, the nail should then be removed by a doctor. If you do not seek treatment, the blood will dry and provide a good culture medium for bacterial or fungal infection. This is usually how a fungal infection of the toenail starts, and once started it can be a time-consuming process eliminating the fungus. As a precautionary measure, keep your toenails short.

If your nails are of the type that tend to be incurvated (curved at the edges), thereby creating ingrown nail problems, cut them squarely so the edges are extending beyond the skin of the toe. If you do not have chronic ingrown toenail problems, then you can trim your nails to fit the curvature of your toe.

Ingrown toenails usually result from the edge of an uncut nail growing and digging into the end of the toe. Besides obvious discomfort, there is a possibility of bacterial infection; if left untreated it can be life-threatening. To treat the toe, the podiatrist will anesthetize it, remove the nail spicule, apply a dressing and give advice as to the proper way to trim your nails. If you have a chronic ingrown toenail problem, minor surgery may be recommended to permanently remove that edge of the nail, usually approximately two millimeters. The procedure is quick, and can be done in the doctor's office.

If you see a black streak, numerous black spots, punctate or punched out areas of the nail, you should consult your doctor immediately. These could be signs of a serious problem.

A subungual exostosis is a bone spur underneath a toenail, usually the biggest one. It is usually marked by severe pain under the toenail, especially when pressure is applied to the top of the nail. Sometimes this bone spur can cause the toenail to lift from its bed and curve inward, thereby contributing to ingrown toenail problems. This is why some doctors will want to X-ray your toe when you have an ingrown toenail. The bone spur treatment consists of minor office surgery; the toe is anesthetized, an incision is made in the tip of the toe, and the bone spur is smoothed down by using a burr.

Mycotic toenails are nails that have fungus in them, which can appear as a gray or white area, streaks in the nail, or nails that are extremely thick, yellow, brown and long; they are called ram's head nails. These will be discussed in the next section.

FUNGAL INFECTIONS

Epidermophyton floccosum, Candida albicans, and a species of Trichophyton are not titles of the latest science fiction books or names of some exotic diseases; rather, they are the types of fungi found on our bodies at all times. These fungi, when they become pathological, are commonly lumped together and known as athlete's foot. Almost every runner will be faced with treating this condition, which causes itching, peeling, redness, and even cracks or fissures in the skin. Fortunately, early treatment of a fungal infection will bring quick improvement just by using an over-the-counter antifungal medication.

Athelete's foot is not restricted to athletes. Any time the skin is restricted for prolonged periods to dark, moist surroundings, the fungus can proliferate.

Athlete's foot, although usually innocuous and easily treated, can become bad enough to require hospitalization, should bacterial infection occur. This is often identified by skin that develops cracks. We have seen patients with swollen feet, peeling skin, red streaks coursing up the legs, and a white, cheesy appearance to different portions of the feet. The patient experiences considerable pain and discomfort. Fortunately this is a rare occurrence, but we mention this to stress the need to treat a minor problem immediately. Also, many people will have dry, peeling skin on the bottoms of their feet; not realizing that this is caused by fungus, they will mistakenly treat it with softening lotions, when they should be using an antifungal cream. For fungal infection, the doctor can administer a simple test in his office by scraping a small amount of the dry skin and putting it in a culture medium.

As mentioned previously, fungus can also invade the toenail. This occurs most often after a traumatic injury, such as a stubbed toe or a partially avulsed nail. A few weeks to a few months later a small gray or white area may be seen on the edge or corners of the nail. With time this portion will enlarge, until the entire nail turns gray. Then the nail will begin to thicken, become extremely hard to cut and may turn yellow. Eventually, some or all the nails might become infected and thickened with fungus or, as is known in medicine, mycotic infection.

Treatment calls for removing the toenail. After a week to ten days, when the nail bed has healed, you will brush the nail bed daily with a toothbrush, which acts as a debriding factor. An antifungal cream is also applied three times a day as the nail grows out. In severe cases, a person can concurrently take an oral antifungal medication, which attacks the infection from inside the body. This may require a monthly blood test to keep track of blood and/or liver parameters. Obviously, you want to recognize athlete's foot symptoms early, when an application of antifungal cream will usually clear up the problem quickly.

BLISTERS

Blisters are a common hazard of anyone who uses his hands or feet for any form of exercise, whether it be gardening or running. Their formation is caused by friction. Constant friction on the skin will separate its many layers. Between these layers fluid enters, which originates from the tissue cells. If friction continues and more skin separates, the blister will enlarge and become more painful. The pain is the result of nerve endings beneath the skin being irritated.

Treatment of a small blister can call for no more than a small aperature pad to take pressure off of it, or, in severe cases — when the entire bottom of the foot is a giant blister — require hospitalization. Preventive measures are encouraged to avoid blisters. If you are susceptible to blistering in a certain part of the foot, the best preventive medicine is to apply to that area a lubricant like Vaseline. Dr. John Pagliano, a sportsmedicine podiatrist in Southern California, recommends applying a handful of Vaseline to the forefoot prior to running a marathon. Also, many athletic shoes have innersole material, which tends to cause blisters more readily than other material. When we buy a pair of athletic shoes, if Spenco is not utilized for the innersole, we will take out the innersole the shoe comes with and put in Spenco. Spenco, being a closed-cell material, allows for lateral shear or movement, plus cushioning. It will also retain its shape and not flatten out.

To treat a blister that has formed and is quite painful, you must first remove fluid underneath the skin. Using an antiseptic solution such as Betadine or just soap and water, cleanse the area well. Then, using a sterile needle or scissors, puncture or cut a small hole in the skin overlying the liquid, allowing the fluid to escape.

Make sure the hole is large enough so that the skin does not close and allow fluid to build up again. Do not remove the overlying skin once the liquid has drained; the underlying skin is too tender to have any pressure or friction on it at this time. Make the following applications: a topical antibiotic to the area of the puncture, an aperture pad to surround the blister and take pressure off of the area, a dressing and tape or Band-Aid. Keep the foot dry for a couple days to prevent a bacterial infection. After a few days, the overlying skin can be removed, again using sterile scissors. If the underlying skin is still tender, an application of moleskin will provide comfort until the skin toughens up.

There are many over-the-counter products that can help prevent blisters, such as Second Skin or New Skin. Wearing thick socks, two layers of socks, the proper size of shoes and using Vaseline are also alternatives. If you feel a hot spot on the bottom of your foot while running, you can be sure a blister is forming. That is the time to stop and take care of your foot.

CORNS

The word corn is a catch-all term referring to a thickening of the skin between and around the toes. There is a distinct difference between corns and calluses, which will be discussed in the next section.

There are two basic types of corns; one is called a heloma durum, which means hard corn, and is usually on the top, bottom or tips of the toes. The other type is known as a heloma molle, which is a soft corn, and is usually between the toes. It is soft because of moisture that is usually present between the toes.

Corns are generally caused by enlargement of the bones in the toes, or from tight-fitting shoes. Either way, an underlying bone rubbing against the shoe or another toe creates a pressure point. The body adapts by thickening the skin to act as a buffer in that pressure area. As this skin thickens with more dead skin cells, the lesion gradually becomes more painful. There is chance of infection, especially from a soft corn between the toes. Early treatment calls for buying wider or larger shoes; a severe corn may require surgery to remove the underlying bone spur or skin enlargement. Before resorting to an operation, other methods are used, such as debriding or trimming down the hyperkeratotic or corn tissue. This usually brings instant relief. The use of an aperture pad or foam tubing applied to the toe usually will prevent the corn from growing back. If conservative treatment does not work, minor surgery is next; it can be done in the office under a local anesthetic.

CALLUSES

A callus or tyloma is different from a corn because it generally occurs on the bottom or the sides of the foot as the result of a pressure from shearing or twisting. Calluses can be as painful as corns, especially if a deep core builds up. There are various degrees and stages of callus development, from a small tyloma − a thickening of the skin on the bottom of the foot − to a nucleated shearing tyloma with a painful core.

Calluses generally have three causes: overpronation, which creates excessive movement in the forefoot when walking; a metatarsal bone, which may be depressed or on a lower plane than the other metatarsals; or another prominent bone on the bottom or the sides of the foot.

Calluses are treated much like corns and blisters; aperature pads are applied after the callus is trimmed. Spenco is used to reduce shearing forces and orthotics will correct excessive pronation. Surgery can be done to raise a depressed metatarsal head to the level of the others, or to remove an enlarged bone elsewhere on the foot.

Calluses most commonly form on the bottom of the forefoot or on the side of the first metatarsal phalangeal joint or big toe. Once the underlying etiology is removed, calluses will likely clear up without further treatment.

WARTS

Warts are commonly mistaken for corns or calluses, especially those on the bottom of the foot. There are two kinds of warts: those that grow on top of the foot, which tend to mushroom out, and those that grow on the bottom of the foot and get pressed into it. The latter are known as plantar (meaning bottom of the foot) warts. Plantar warts usually have hyperkeratotic or callous material overlying them. Upon debriding the callous material, you will see a cheesy-looking growth with small, black dots in the center of the lobes. These are the blood vessels and nerves growing in the virus material. There is also more pain on lateral palpation or pinching than on direct pressure.

Because warts are a virus material, some people are more prone than others to having them. They often start while a person has a small cut on the bottom of the foot; the cut provides a portal of entry for the virus. If the virus is not treated within a short time, it will begin spreading to other areas of the foot. In very severe cases it can cover the bottom of the entire foot or both feet; this is known as a mosaic wart. It is also possible to infect other members of the family.

Treatment claims abound: garlic around the neck, hypnotism, and so on. But they can clear up spontaneously, so don't be fooled if one of these exotic treatments works. The usual treatment is by one of several methods, such as currettage (numbing the area and scooping out the lesion), fulgeration (burning the wart with an electrode), repetitive acid treatments, and surgical excision. Newer, promising treatments are utilizing cancer chemotherapy injections.

A frequent recommendation is weekly applications of 60 percent salicylic acid. The wart is debrided, an aperature pad is put on to surround the wart, and a small amount of salicylic acid, usually in a cream base, is applied with a dressing that overlies it. The foot is kept dry, and once a week the wart material is debrided. Salicylic acid is applied until it has disappeared. Other methods work well, but there is the possibility that scar tissue may develop, whereas with salicylic acid there is no scaring. Obviously, a doctor can make the best choice of treatment.

HAMMERTOES

A hammertoe is a toe that is cocked up. It is usually caused by the tendons holding the toe in a constant state of contracture. Many times the problem is hereditary, but almost always you will find an overpronated foot creating the hammertoe. Generally, they are not painful and cause no problems, as long as the proper shoes, such as those with large toe boxes, are worn.

To complicate matters, corns can form on the top of the hammertoe, or calluses under the metatarsal head. This is the result of a retrograde force on the metatarsal head from the cocked toe. Other problems are corns at the tip of the toe, from the tip resting on the ground, and also toenail problems, such as partial tearing of the nail from socks getting caught beneath the nail.

You can have a rigid or flexible hammertoe. The flexible hammertoe usually can be corrected by eliminating pronation through the utilization of orthotics. The rigid hammertoe can only be corrected through surgery. A portion of the toe bone is removed, and in some cases the tendon is lengthened, thereby allowing the toe to lay flat. Conservative treatment calls for a crest pad underlying the toe, and accommodating the corns and calluses by using pads, foam tubing, lamb's wool, etc.

MORTON'S TOE

Morton's toe or Morton's foot, as it's called, is seen as an extra-long second toe. It was mentioned as a sign of intelligence in Greek literature. Today we know Morton's toe has nothing to do with intelligence and that it is the source of a myriad of foot problems.

The long second toe is either caused by a shortened first metatarsal or an elongated second metatarsal. Either one of these two conditions usually causes a hypermobile first metatarsal and big toe. Together they are known as the first ray. The condition allows excessive pronation and undue pressure under the second metatarsal head. Pain under the second metatarsal head is one of the common problems associated with a Morton's toe. It is possible to shorten the long second metatarsal, but the problem is usually a short first metatarsal. Orthotics, which will control over-pronation, will take care of any related problems. Usually the orthotic will have a first metatarsal extension to support the first metatarsal head.

BUNIONS

We are going to dispel a common misconception: Paul Bunyan was not a podiatrist. What he may have had, though, was a large bump on the inside of the foot at the base of the big toe joint. This bump is commonly called a bunion.

There is a large tendon attached to the inside of the big toe. As the foot overpronates, this tendon is stretched and begins pulling the big toe toward the other toes. A retrograde force of the big toe against the first metatarsal pushes the head of the bone toward the medial or inside of the foot. This marks the beginning of the bump. Continual pressure from shoe gear, etc., on the medial side of the head of the first metatarsal causes more bone to be layed down there as a protective mechanism. Like the callus, this is a self-defeating situation. As the big toe drifts further toward the other toes, the cartilage in the first metatarsal phalangeal joint begins to erode. Eventually the cartilage becomes completely eroded and you have bone rubbing on bone — very painful. Other forces that come into play are the big toe underriding the second toe. It becomes hammered, creating retrograde force on the second metatarsal head; the problems keep compounding themselves. The big toe can become severely deviated.

Bunions may be hereditary or they can develop over time because of overpronation. But even if a person has a bunion resulting from heredity, he generally will also have an overpronated foot. This hallux valgus with bunion deformity, as it is called by podiatrists, can make difficult finding proper-fitting shoes. The bunion is unsightly and the joint is prone to traumatic arthritis. Also, the two little bones beneath the big toe joint, or the first metatarsal phalangeal joint, called sesamoids, become irritated. These two round bones protect the flexor tendon as it goes beneath the joint. As the hallux valgus deformity worsens, the sesamoid bones can also become painful.

Treatment is twofold: First, you must remove the forces creating the problem — deformity and overpronation. Orthotics will correct excessive pronation, and surgery is needed to eliminate the deformity. Strapping, padding or orthotics alone will not correct the deformity. There are many types of surgical procedures, or bunionectomies, and each case has to be reviewed individually.

At the base of the fifth toe you can also have a bump, which is called a tailor's bunion. It is sometimes referred to as bunionette. The term tailor's bunion has an interesting origin. It was named after tailors, who would sit cross-legged for long hours, which would create pressure on the head of the fifth metatarsal. A bump ensued. Orthotics will not alleviate this problem, and if padding does not relieve the discomfort, minor surgery to remove the bump is indicated. Treat your bunions as soon as possible. The longer you wait, the more extensive will be the corrective procedure.

STRESS FRACTURES

We include stress fractures here because the metatarsal bones are commonly the ones affected by the stresses of sports, especially running. But we do see stress fractures in other bones, especially the lower fibula and midshaft tibia.

The cause of stress fractures is essentially the same. It can be an overt fracture, caused by excessive stress on the bone, but then again any type of fracture will fit that description. We are going to discuss the type of fracture that causes pain, but shows no bone abnormality on an X-ray, at least at the onset of the fracture. The following case study will give you some idea how a stress fracture can occur, and its symptoms.

Nancy was training for the San Francisco Marathon. One day after a run she noticed pain in the middle of her forefoot. Thinking this to be strained ligaments or muscles, she layed off running for a couple of days; she had no pain while walking. She began running again after three days. But after a half mile the same pain returned and prevented her from continuing her run. She visited our office for treatment. X-rays showed no fracture. But because the pain on palpation (applying pressure with hands) was approximately midshaft of the second metatarsal, we made a tentative diagnosis of stress fracture. Nancy was instructed to not run for three weeks and to return to the office at that time for a follow-up X-ray. The X-ray taken three weeks later revealed signs of a fracture on the shaft of the second metatarsal. The preliminary, tentative diagnosis of stress fracture was confirmed. Nancy was advised to not run for another week, and that she should resume training at a reduced rate. Since her training was disrupted, she opted to run the Honolulu Marathon, which was five months later than the San Francisco Marathon.

Why did the X-ray show no fracture the first time? Because the microscopic break in the cortex, the outer layer of the bone, cannot be picked up on an X-ray. The body begins to lay calcium around the area of the stress fracture to heal and strengthen the bone. It takes approximately three to four weeks for enough calcium to be layed down for it to show up on an X-ray. That's why a follow-up X-ray was done one month later. Usually the person is back running by the time the calcium or bone callus, as it is called, can be seen on an X-ray.

NERVE TUMORS

The most common type of nerve tumor in the foot is called a neuroma. This is a benign nerve tumor commonly appearing between the third and fourth metatarsal heads.

A neuroma can occur anywhere in the foot where there is irritation to the nerve sheath. This irritation causes a thickening of the sheath, which in turn causes more irritation. Symptoms include a needle-piercing pain that "shoots" out into the toes, tingling, numbness, or muscle cramping.

Treatment for a neuroma consists of removing the pressure against the nerve. Neuromas, which are usually caused by an over-pronated foot, can be relieved by wearing orthotics. Orthotics help separate the metatarsal heads. Other remedies include padding the area between the metatarsal heads, steroid injections and anti-inflammatory medications. If conservative therapy does not elim-inate the problem, surgery is called for. The tumor can be removed in the office, under local anesthetic. Since this is soft-tissue sur-gery, recovery is not so long as with bone surgery. Walking the same day as surgery and normal running within a couple weeks is routine. Other common locations for neuromas are on the top of the foot and on the side of the heel.

CYSTS

Cysts can be felt on the foot as small, usually movable, bumps beneath the skin. They are outpouchings or herniations of tendon sheaths or joint capsules. These herniations fill with a clear, gela-tinous fluid. They are usually not painful, although when they lie near a nerve, pressure against the nerve may create discomfort. Cysts are benign, but any lump on the foot should be examined by a doctor.

Grandma's tactic for treating ganglionic cysts was to take a large book and give the cyst a good whack, which would rupture the herniated sack. Although this is not recommended, it did oc-casionally work.

Treatment is unnecessary if the cyst is not irritating you. You may need to relieve pressure caused by wearing shoes, or have it drained. The gelatinous fluid is removed with a large bore needle and syringe. Again, all lumps, bumps or growths on the foot should be checked by a podiatrist as soon as possible.

6

Rearfoot Injuries

Injuries to the rear of the foot tend to be less common than forefoot injuries. But they do afflict every age group and result from a variety of sports activities. Nor are they discriminatory as to sex.

PAIN IN THE BOTTOM OF THE FOOT

Refer to Fig. 6-1. There is a very thick, fibrous band of tissue that runs along the bottom of the foot, called the plantar fascia. It attaches to the heel on the bottom, extends forward into the foot and spreads out into four separate bands that attach to the toe webs. This band of tissue is so thick and fibrous that it has no elasticity. The function of the plantar fascia is to help support the foot — along with other structures — and to form the arch. The fascia is most commonly injured or torn in the middle of the arch and at the attachment to the heel bone. This heel injury is known as a heel spur syndrome.

Tearing or rupturing the ligamentous fibers is usually caused by a stretched or strained plantar fascia, the result of repetitive over-pronation, excessive upward bending of the foot or toes, or a bruise.

Pain is usually low-grade — a persistent nagging that might last for months, even years. Usually the pain is more acute in the morning or after strenuous exercise. The first step in the morning

49

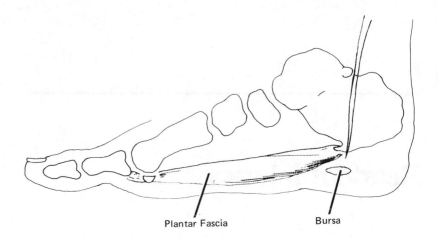

Plantar Fascia   Bursa

Fig. 6-1

when getting out of bed might be excruciatingly painful; discomfort lessens with walking, only to return later in the day.

Treatment calls for resting the ligamentous band and reducing any tension you might normally place on it. This can be done by taping the foot with a low-dye strapping, using felt varus wedges or orthotics; in extreme cases the foot is put in a cast for a couple of weeks. Heat, from a steam pack or ultrasound, will promote blood flow into the thick, fibrous tissue. We have found that the combination of orthotics and ultrasound is the best treatment for plantar fasciitis.

HEEL PAIN

If you have just turned to this page to find out why you have pain on the bottom of the heel, we recommend that you first read the previous section on plantar fasciitis. Pain on the bottom of the heel is usually caused by inflammation of the plantar fascia at the attachment to the bottom of the heel. The etiology is generally the same — overpronation or trauma. X-rays may reveal a large bone spur on the bottom of the heel, extending toward the front of the foot. Surprisingly, pain in the plantar fascia is not from the bone spur, but rather the inflammation encountered where the ligament attaches to the bone. Inflammation causes cells to migrate to the area; some of these cells are bone-laying cells. What ensues is a bone spur in the area of the inflammation; over a period of several years, the bone spur can become quite long. But the spur is a secondary finding and not the cause of the pain. It is the pull of the plantar fascia away from the heel bone that is source of the problem. A long run, soft shoes, running on an uneven road, or a blow to the area — all of these can lead to plantar fasciitis.

Treatment, as mentioned, consists of taking tension off of the plantar fascia where it attaches to the heel. It may be in the form of taping, wedges, harder-soled shoes, orthotics, heat (steam pack or ultrasound) and injections of a local anesthetic and a steroid. Injections work well; they reduce inflammation quickly, but the forces causing the heel pain also have to be removed to prevent its return. Surgery may be called for to detach the ligament from the heel — at which time the bone spur can also be removed — but surgery is rarely done. We have successfully treated more than 99 percent of our patients with heel-spur problems using conservative, non-surgical methods.

Back of heel: Please refer to Fig. 6-1. Notice that the Achilles tendon attaches to the back of the heel. Between the tendon and the bone is a small, fluid-filled sack called a bursa. Think of it as a ball bearing that sits between the tendon and the bone, and prevents the tendon from becoming inflamed. However, constant friction, from a tight shoe pressing on the skin and the tendon for example, can cause the bursa to become inflamed; this creates what is called a retro calcaneal bursitis. Occasionally the Achilles tendon will also become inflamed. You may have seen large bumps on some people's heels. These were quite common in the 1950s when women wore pumps. This condition became known as a "pump bump."

Through chronic inflammation, the bursal sack can calcify, causing a prominent and painful bump on the back of the heel. Once there is calcification, the usual treatment is surgery to remove the bump. Non-surgical treatment consists of padding the bump until the inflammation subsides, injections with a local anesthetic and a steroid, ice, aspirin or other anti-inflammatory medications, and in severe cases a cast to eliminate foot movement so the bursa and/or the Achilles tendinitis can heal.

Calcaneal apophysitis: Apophysitis means inflammation of the growth area of the calcaneus or heel bone. This is generally seen in those between the age of ten and fifteen. The accompanying pain can be in the back of the heel or beneath it, and the area is most painful when it is squeezed.

We often see calcaneal apophysitis in youngsters who are involved in sports with considerable running and jumping, such as basketball, baseball and soccer. The spiked shoes that are worn in the latter two sports can usually be blamed for apophysitis on the bottom of the heel. Treatment consists of half-inch felt lifts to be placed in both shoes and/or a heel cup. X-rays are necessary to determine if there has been a fracture of the growth area.

Activity must be restricted for a few weeks; this can be an extremely frustrating injury for an active, growing youngster, but fortunately it clears up without sequela.

PAIN ON THE INSIDE OF THE FOOT

Pain on the inside of the foot can result from a host of reasons. First, a quick review of its anatomy is in order (see Figs. 1-5, 1-6). Notice where the posterior tibial tendon comes down along the inside of the foot and attaches to the medial or inside aspect of the navicular bone. This area of attachment is a common source of pain experienced on the side of the foot. The pain can be the result of posterior tibial tendinitis, an enlarged navicular, a fractured navicular, or an accessory navicular bone.

Posterior tibial tendinitis usually develops when feet prone to excessive pronation are put in soft-soled shoes. The attachment of the tendon on the navicular becomes partially torn, and inflammation results; the discomfort can be compared to a needle- or knife-like pain. Treatment consists of removing overpronation with orthotics or harder-soled shoes and physical therapy to reduce the discomfort.

If you have an enlarged navicular and a foot or feet that overpronate, the bone can rub against the side of the shoe, or in severe cases the navicular bone may hit the opposite inside ankle bone as the foot is swinging forward. If non-surgical treatment — padding or orthotics — does not eliminate the problem, surgery is recommended to remove the enlarged portion.

Because the area of the navicular near the attachment of the tendon is also a growth plate area, non-fusion of the growth plate sometimes results. You will develop what is called an accessory navicular. The result of non-union and the tendon constantly tugging in this area is discomfort. There is not enough support for the tendon. The problem is usually solved by using orthotics. Pain on the inside of the foot could also be caused by a ligament strain, trauma, stress fracture, nerve tumor, etc. That's why a doctor should make the diagnosis.

PAIN ON THE TOP OF THE FOOT

Pain or discomfort on the top of the foot is usually caused by tendinitis and/or bone spurs at the joints of the foot. Also, a high arch will cause the joints to jam, which can create discomfort; but most problems here come from the low-arched or overpronated foot. Bend your toes up and see the many tendons attached to them; they traverse the top of the foot and extend up into the ankle. These tendons are used when the foot is in the swing phase of gait and to decelerate the toes prior to forefoot contact. If you switch to shoes with a higher heel or do a lot of downhill running, these tendons can be stretched and aggravated; tendinitis results. Other causes include shoes that are laced too tight and eyelets that are too large. Or the tongue of a shoe might get crimped and cause intense pressure on the top of the foot. That was what forced Dr. Zamzow out of the California Road Runners 100-Mile Endurance Run in 1981, with only ten miles to go.

Bone spurs can form at the top of the joints in the foot because of a very low arch. Continual jamming of a joint can cause a portion of the top part of the bone to break off, thus starting spur formation. In some cases, these spurs are quite large, painful bumps that make wearing shoes almost impossible.

Tendinitis is treated with aspirin, ice — if there is swelling — heat (after a few days) and rest. The cause of the tendinitis must be found to be eliminated.

Other ailments include gangleonic cysts, nerve tumors, pinched nerves, and bone spurs on the top of the talus neck; the spurs jam into the front of the tibia or leg bone and cause discomfort.

PAIN ON THE OUTSIDE OF THE FOOT

Pain on the outside of the foot has three major causes: peroneal muscle tendinitis, inflammation at the attachment of the peroneal muscle tendon to the fifth metatarsal base (see Fig. 6-2), and ligament strain.

The forces creating peroneal tendinitis can sometimes be difficult to track down and eliminate. This is a rather rare injury,

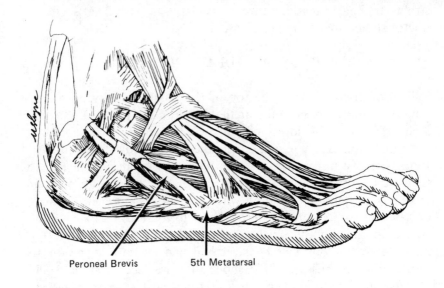

Peroneal Brevis   5th Metatarsal

Fig. 6-2   Lateral Foot

and although the tendinitis can clear up, it may take several tries at changing shoes, terrain, sports, gait, and rest.

An enlarged fifth metatarsal base pressing against the side of a shoe can cause considerable discomfort. Padding to accommodate the metatarsal will eliminate the pain, and rarely is surgery necessary.

High-arched feet generally cause trouble on the outside of the foot. Their inability to absorb shock makes them difficult to treat, whereas the flatfooted person is easier to treat. Dr. George Sheehan refers to the high-arched foot as "clunk foot." We have found that the best way to neutralize the high arch is to prescribe a flexible sport orthotic. The flexible orthotic acts as a shock absorber for the foot. Also, well-cushioned shoes are advised for the clunk foot.

7

Ankle Injuries

As discussed in Chapter 1, the ankle joint serves as the connection between the foot and the leg. Review Fig. 1-9 ; note the two bones that come down from the leg — the tibia and the fibula, respectively, and how they connect to the foot vis-a-vis the ankle. The ankle joint has only two directions of motion in a single plane, up and down. These motions are known as dorsiflexion and plantarflexion, as shown in Fig. 1-10a, b. Even though the ankle joint functions in just one plane of motion, it is one of the most important joints in the body because it must smoothly operate as the connector between the foot and leg at each step.

Fig. 7-1a shows the main structures that hold the ankle joint together. On the inside is the deltoid ligament. This large band consists of four individual components that coalesce into one large ligament. The deltoid ligament fans out from the tip of the tibia and inserts into four separate bones of the foot. This is a very important point to remember when considering the ankle injuries discussed later.

The outside of the ankle joint, by comparison, is very weak. As shown in Fig. 7-1b, there are three separate, small ligaments that make up the outside connection between the foot and ankle. Note the names, which are derived from where the ligaments originate and attach. These three small ligaments have the job of maintaining ankle stability — a job which, unfortunately, they are ill-suited to perform. When injury occurs, these ligaments are more

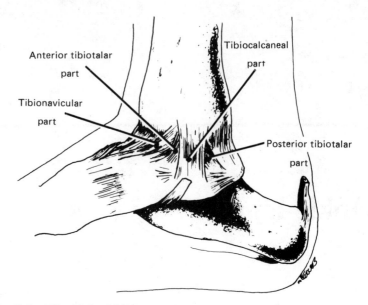

Fig. 7-1a The Deltoid Ligament.

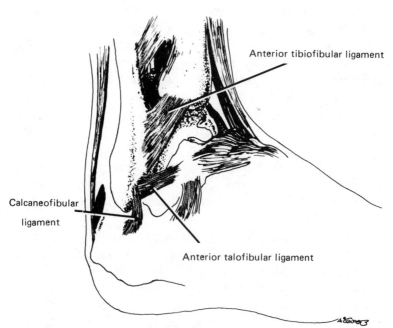

Fig. 7-1b The Lateral Ankle

vulnerable to damage than the ligaments on the inside of the ankle, the deltoid.

In addition to these main ligaments mentioned, there are several other structures that contribute to ankle stability. The majority of ankle strength comes from the tendons that cross it. The muscles that originate from the lower leg send out tendons to the foot, which cross both the front, back and both sides of the ankle. But despite all the structures that attempt to hold the ankle joint tightly together, this joint is prone to injury. Moreover, injuries to the ankle joint tend to be more serious and lasting than injuries to other joints.

INJURIES

In this section we will not be discussing major fractures of the bones in and around the ankle. These injuries are caused by a direct blow to the area; there is usually major displacement of the ankle bones. These injuries require immediate medical attention and in extreme cases surgery may be required in order to pin or screw the various fractured bones together. More common, and our topic of discussion, are ankle sprains or overuse injuries where there may be a small, nondisplaced bone break or damage to the ligaments or tendons, or both.

The most common ankle injury — more common than all others combined — is called an inversion sprain. The structure of the leg and foot, for technical reasons, make the ankle prone to this type of injury. An inversion sprain occurs when the foot is suddenly twisted in the direction as shown in Fig. 7-2. This can occur by stepping off a curb wrong, tripping over a rock, and so on. As discussed in Chapter 2, the foot is designed to function with a limited amount of motion in the direction of inversion (also known as supination). However, in an inversion sprain the foot is overstressed in the direction of supination and reaches its maximum end range of motion; in other words, it can no longer normally go any farther. But with an inversion sprain, because the foot is forced past its end range of motion, something must give.

If the injury is mild, the ligaments and the tendons around the ankle will absorb the added stress with either minimal or no damage. Recovery from a mild sprain occurs within several minutes; there is no pain, swelling or residual damage.

The more severe inversion sprain is a different story. The stress, that is generated as the foot travels past its maximum range of

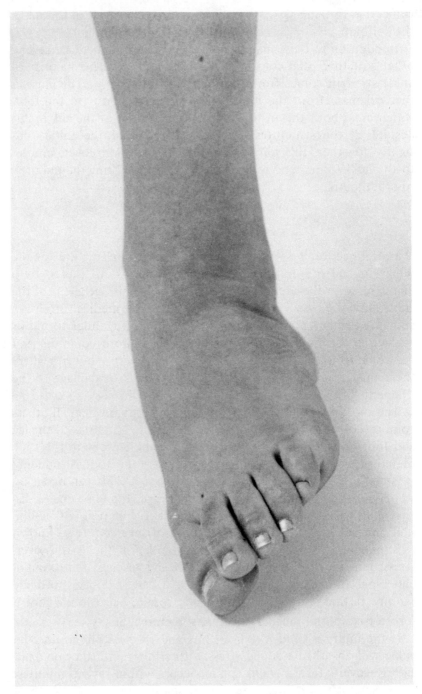

Fig. 7-2 *Inversion sprains—the most common of ankle injuries— occur when the foot is suddenly twisted in the direction shown here.*

supination is too great for the ligaments and tendons to withstand. As a result, the brunt of the damage is taken by the three small ligaments on the outside of the ankle. When injury occurs, these ligaments are immediately stressed to the point that either a pull or tear occurs.

The sequence of ligament damage in all inversion sprains goes like this: The front ligament, the anterior talofibular ligament, always takes the majority of the initial stress, and this is the first to be torn or pulled. If the foot stops its motion at this point, this will be the only ligament that is damaged. If, however, the foot keeps going, the ligament that runs from the tip of the fibula to the heel bone (see Fig. 1-3) will snap next. And if the foot continues inverting, the rear ligament also tears. This type of sprain, where all three ligaments tear, is severe and uncommon. Typically, in even a mild sprain, the front ligament is injured.

TENDON INJURY IN AN INVERSION SPRAIN

The peroneal tendons run down the outside of the leg, attaching to the foot in two different places (see Fig. 7-3). These tendons evert the foot. Therefore, in an inversion sprain, they are stretched. In a mild strain these tendons have enough elasticity to withstand the load, or some of the tendon fibers will be torn and lead to a tendinitis. If the sprain is moderate to severe, however, these tendons must give at some point along their course. The peroneal brevis tendon, in this case, pulls so suddenly that it yanks off the bone where it attaches to the foot, as shown in Fig. 7-3. This is known as a Jones fracture and calls for professional treatment.

Treatment

Inversion sprains, or for that matter any ankle sprain, must be treated with respect. Any injury to the ligaments around the ankle joint, if not properly treated, can lead to permanent ankle instability. If another sprain should occur, the debilitated ligaments will not be able to take up the strain. This situation allows for damage to the bones of the ankle joint to occur, which might result in permanent disability and arthritis. So all ankle injuries, no matter how small, should be treated immediately.

At the outset of the injury do the following: 1) Stop all further activity no matter how minor the injury may appear. A minor pain can get worse if exercise is continued; serious damage might occur. 2) Re-create the injury in your mind. Exactly how was the foot

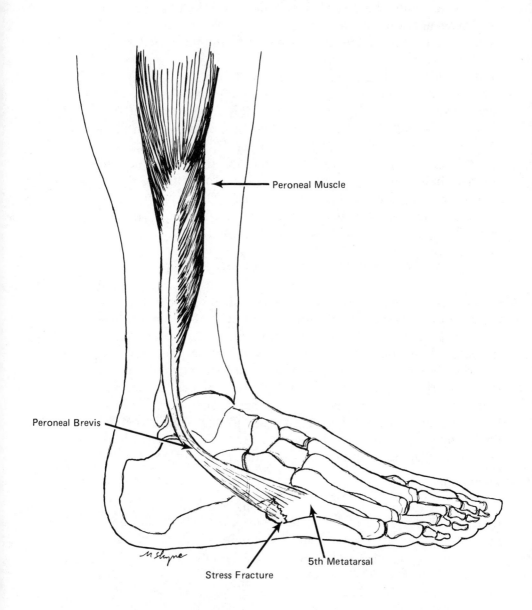

Fig. 7-3   Jones Fracture

turned? Did you hear or feel a crunch or pop? This information will help a physician make a diagnosis.

Self-Treatment

Begin self-treatment immediately after the injury. A clever nomic has been devised to cover the immediate phase of the injury —R.I.C.E., which stands for rest, ice, compression and elevation. Proper self-treatment begins here.

We'll go through the four treatments and explain their benefits. Rest is vital after an injury, no matter how minor. The body needs time to concentrate on repairing the damage. Start with ice immediately following the injury and for several days afterward. Ice constricts the blood vessels in the damaged area and thus reduces swelling. Compression serves two purposes. First, compression — done by squeezing on the injured area — prevents excessive swelling. Second, and perhaps more important, compression immobilizes the area. Immobilization is desired to reduce the risk of further injury. Elevation will also reduce swelling and pain by preventing blood from pooling at the injury. The healing process is enhanced by following these four treatments. Furthermore, when you seek professional help these four points are the cornerstone of the treatment plan that will get you healthy and back to your activity.

After a few minutes of icing, evaluate the injury. There will no doubt be swelling. But this is normal. The amount of swelling is not the determining factor as to the extent of injury. We have seen horribly swollen injured ankles after an injury that were not fractured. Conversely, we have seen ankle injuries with minimal swelling, but that had two or three separate breaks within the joint.

Also, a black-and-blue bruise will be noticed around the ankle. This indicates that tissue damage and hence a rupture of small blood vessels has occurred. By palpating (touching) a couple of important points on the foot and ankle, the severity of the injury can be determined.

First, examine the area around the styloid process of the fifth metatarsal to determine if a Jones fracture, as shown in Fig. 7-3, has occurred. If, on pressing lightly around this area, it is even mildly painful suspect a fracture and get immediate medical attention. Next, examine the anterior tibiofibular ligament located in the front of the ankle, as was shown in Fig. 1-3. Again, if the area is tender or there is a sharp pain in this area consider the ligament to be severly injured. Also palpate the other ligaments to see if these are tender. If they are, the injury is serious. Furthermore, if you

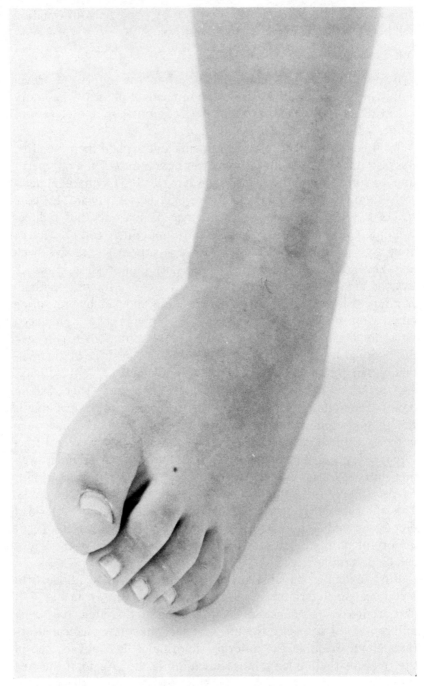

Fig. 7-4 *The foot in an everted position.*

are unable to walk without pain several minutes after the injury, damage has occurred. If any one or all of these self-tests are positive, get medical attention.

If a ligament is torn and does not heal properly, it cannot effectively carry out its function of stability. Ligaments, in order to heal properly, must be immobilized. Therefore, if we suspect any degree of ligament damage, we apply a below-the-knee walking cast or, in mild cases, with an Ace bandage and crutches. We have seen many injured athletes who have ignored ankle sprains and have suffered permanent, irreversible damage as a result.

Other, less common sprains, can occur through eversion. As shown in Fig. 7-4, the foot is being turned in an everted position. Because the deltoid ligament is large and strong in comparison to the ligaments on the outside of the ankle, eversion injuries will more likely cause a bone to break than tear a ligament. Eversion sprains are generally more painful than inversion sprains, and deserve immediate medical attention. Common injuries such as tendinitis, bursitis or bone spurs can also occur around the ankle joint.

8

The Leg

We are discussing problems encountered in the leg because they affect your gait cycle, thereby creating unique functional problems for the foot. Look at Fig. 8-1; notice that the leg is divided into four compartments, separated by non-elastic sheaths. The sheath in itself can produce problems, which will be discussed here.

PAIN AT THE FRONT OF THE LEG

Generally, pain at the front of the leg can be attributed to two causes: either an anterior tibial muscle strain, commonly known as shinsplints, or a stress fracture in the anterior or front portion of the tibia bone.

The symptom of shinsplints is noticed as a very sharp pain in the anterior muscle group while running, and especially while running downhill. The root cause is that the anterior muscles are not as strong as the posterior muscles — calf muscles or gastrocnemius soleus complex — and therefore fatigue sooner. Running strengthens the calf muscles, quadriceps muscles, and back muscles considerably more so than the anterior leg, posterior thigh, or abdominal muscles. The calf muscles, being considerably stronger, will have more endurance. Thus, the anterior leg muscle group will fatigue first, with considerable lactic acid buildup, which causes pain. The discomfort is especially noticeable when bending or

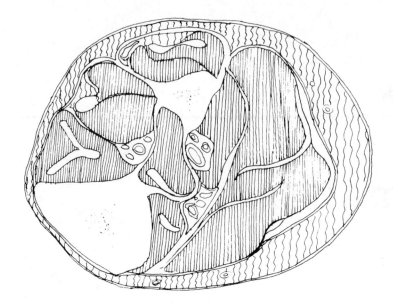

Fig. 8-1 Cross-Section of the Lower Leg

plantarflexing your foot down, and on palpation of the anterior tibial muscle group.

Treatment is aimed at relieving the inflammation via heat, deep tissue massage and anti-inflammatory medication. Once the inflammation clears up, the anterior muscle group should be strengthened to eliminate the disparity in strength and endurance between the anterior and posterior muscles. Here's a simple exercise to work the anterior muscles: place a weight over the top of the foot (like a paint can) and raise the foot up and down by flexing your ankle in a series of repetitive motions. Perform this two or three times a day for several weeks.

Another uncommon but serious problem that can occur in the anterior muscle group is the compartment syndrome. This is the result of a leg muscle expanding beyond the bounds of its non-elastic compartment sheath. Muscle compression, restriction of blood flow and, in severe cases, necrosis (muscle tissue death) can occur. While rest will usually eliminate the pain, it returns upon resumption of activities. Compartment syndrome is hard to diagnose, but once established, minor surgery will remedy the problem. Basically the compartment fascia is slit, thereby allowing the muscle to expand. Mary Decker and John Walker are notable runners who have had compartment syndrome.

PAIN ON THE INSIDE OF THE LEG

Posterior tibial tendinitis resulting from overpronation is the culprit for most problems on the inside of the leg. Fig. 1-12 shows the posterior tibial muscle originating deep within the leg, where it is attached between the tibia and fibula. The muscle courses to the inside of the leg where the tendon of the posterior tibial muscle follows the tibia around the posterior portion of the medial malleolus or ankle bone, attaching to the navicular. When the foot overpronates from biomechanical abnormalities such as running shoes collapsing to the inside, the cant of the road, and in some cases inflexibility, the posterior tibial muscle fibers develop microscopic tears away from the bone; the tendon's sheath also rubs against the bone where it courses down the leg. Pain and swelling occur. As discussed in Chapter 6 under inside rearfoot problems, a differential diagnosis has to be made between a stress fracture and tendinitis, or myositis, which is muscle inflammation. Generally, a stress fracture will be identified by a pinpoint of tenderness, whereas pain due to posterior tibial tendinitis usually extends down the leg.

Treatment consists of removing the forces of overpronation, via new shoes, running on a level surface and, if necessary, orthotics. Inflammation is reduced by ultrasound, steam packs, deep-tissue massage and, if appropriate, anti-inflammatory medication. Pain on the inside of the leg — specifically, posterior tibial tendinitis — is probably the most common location for leg trouble.

PAIN IN THE BACK OF THE LEG

Fig. 1-6 shows the gastrocnemius soleus muscle complex with its associated tendon inserting at the back of the calcaneus or heel bone. Note that the gastrocnemius originates at two points above the knee in the back of the femur or thigh bone. The soleus' origin is below the knee from the back of the tibia and fibula. They both join and become the Achilles tendon.

Achilles tendinitis is primarily the result of overuse and/or overextension of the tendon. Note in Fig. 8-2 that the Achilles tendon does not have a tendon sheath, as do other tendons. The Achilles tendon is surrounded by a thin covering known as a paratenon, which poorly supplies the tendon with blood. Any injury to the Achilles, therefore, is slow to heal.

In this next scenario, we will illustrate how Achilles tendinitis comes about. A runner gets out of bed in the morning and the first thing he does is some stretching exercises, which may be strenuous or ballistic in nature. He takes off running on a cold morning at a pace that might be too fast and there is a hill in the early part of the run. After his run, he doesn't stretch. The next morning when the runner gets out of bed, he notices his calf muscles and Achilles tendons hurt. Here's what he should have done: Walk or jog slowly for a mile to get the blood circulating; walk up hills in the early part of the run; and do slow, progressive stretching exercises — after warming up in the middle of the run — that are non-ballistic and yoga-like. After the run, walk and stretch. It has been said that three types of runners will generally have Achilles tendon problems: those who run in the morning, those who are heavy, and tall women.

You should not run with Achilles tendon pain. Tendon fibers that have been ripped or strained can possibly worsen and may tear from the heel bone or separate and break in two. That could result in a long post-surgical rehabilitation program requiring a cast for up to six months.

If you notice upon awakening or as the day progresses that there is a creaking feeling in the Achilles tendon, it is definitely time to stop all activities and seek professional help. If this creaking feeling is allowed to continue, which is caused by swelling around the Achilles tendon, scar tissue may develop between the paratenon and the surrounding tissue. Once this scar tissue develops, chronic pain will ensue, which can only be corrected by surgical intervention.

Stretching is important to prevent Achilles tendon problems. We have a simple test that tells you if you have been stretching enough. Lie on the floor with your legs straight and bend your foot up. Measure an angle along the outside of the foot and along a line going up the leg. This should be about 90 degrees. You should then be able to bend your foot toward your face, decreasing the angle to at least 80 degrees. If you do not have this 10 degrees of dorsiflexion with your leg straight, start a stretching program. Now bend your knee, and bend your foot at the ankle. It should bend farther in this position. You will probably be able to get the angle down to 75 or 60 degrees, or a 10- to 15-degree dorsiflexion off of the perpendicular. With the leg bent, the gastrocnemius portion is relaxed, so the soleus muscle's range of motion is being

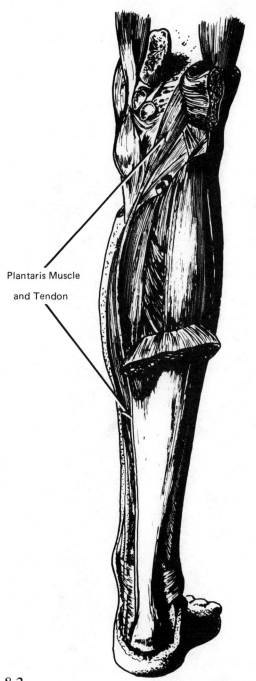

Plantaris Muscle
and Tendon

Fig. 8-2

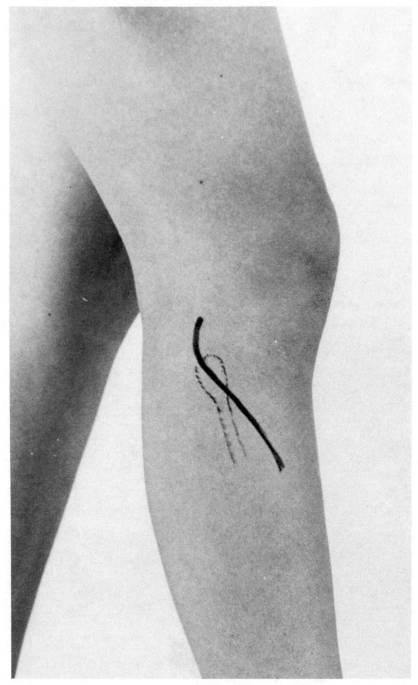

Fig. 8-3 *This photo shows where the peroneal nerve passes over the fibula, directly below the outside of the knee.*

measured. If you can't bend your foot 10 degrees from the perpendicular, you have what is known as an equinus. We recommend you read the self-treatment chapter on stretching.

Fig. 8-2 shows the plantaris muscle with its long tendon running beside the Achilles tendon and inserting into the heel. Occasionally the plantaris can rupture, causing severe pain that mimics Achilles tendinitis.

As you can see, prevention is the key to eliminating posterior leg pain. If problems do develop, rest, heat, deep-tissue massage, ice massage alternating with heat at the Achilles tendon, heel lifts, ultrasound and, as healing occurs, stretching to reduce the chance of future problems may be necessary.

If you have Achilles discomfort when you get up in the morning, apply heat to the area utilizing a steam pack prior to running; jog lightly for the first couple of miles, and end with light stretching followed by ice massage.

PAIN AT THE OUTSIDE OF THE LEG

While pain at the outside of the leg is rare, it is usually caused by two factors: a stress fracture of the fibula, and peroneal muscle tendinitis. At the time of this writing, we have seen less than ten cases of peroneal muscle tendinitis. Most of those patients had high arches. This tendinitis is usually aggravated by the road cant. Running on the cant of a road can also cause strain at the head of the fibula, just below the knee where the fibula joins to the tibia with ligaments. In many cases the result is a ligamentous strain, which can take a couple weeks to heal.

A stress fracture of the fibula is usually in its lower portion. See Fig. 7-3 and also see the discussion on stress fractures in Chapter 5. In fact, a stress fracture of the fibular malleolus is the most common type of stress fracture we see. It usually requires a leg cast.

A word of caution regarding below-the-knee walking casts. Just below the head of the fibula (directly below the outside of the knee), the peroneal nerve courses over the bone and down the side of the leg — see Fig. 8-3. It is not uncommon for the cast to be applied so high that it rubs against this nerve and in some cases permanently damages the nerve, paralyzing the leg muscles and causing what is known as a drop-foot. If you have such a cast applied to your leg, make sure the doctor locates the nerve and has the top portion of the cast start just below it.

The peroneal muscles can become spastic due to a fusion of the talus and calcaneus at the subtalar joint in the foot. This can be congenital or traumatic in origin, and professional help must be sought.

9

The Knee

Why devote a chapter to the knee when this is a book about foot problems? Because the foot has a profound effect on the entire leg-knee-back area. And the knee, because of its unique structure and function, is the most vulnerable joint when acted upon by abnormal foot function. A recent survey of running injuries, published in *Runner's World* magazine, bears this out. Knee injuries were the No. 1 complaint. Almost every active person will suffer from some type of knee injury at one time or another.

We will discuss injuries related to overuse secondary to foot and leg imbalances. Acute knee injury is not our concern here and this problem should be treated by a sportsmedicine orthopedist. Moreover, any injury to the knee and its surrounding structures that causes it to unlock, give out, swell or have limited motion, also requires orthopedic consultation. Typically, knee injuries that occur in such sports as skiing or football are traumatic. We do not imply that these types of severe injuries are caused by foot imbalances, albeit imbalances can contribute to them.

The knee is a complex yet relatively weak joint. Unfortunately, the largest joint in the body is held together by only a few internal structures. Fig. 9-1 shows these structures. Note the collateral ligaments that extend down the inside and outside of the joint. The cruciate ligaments, directly within the joint, criss-cross. The minisci act as cushioning pads between the femur and tibia. In addition to these small ligaments, there are several other less important structures that help support the knee joint.

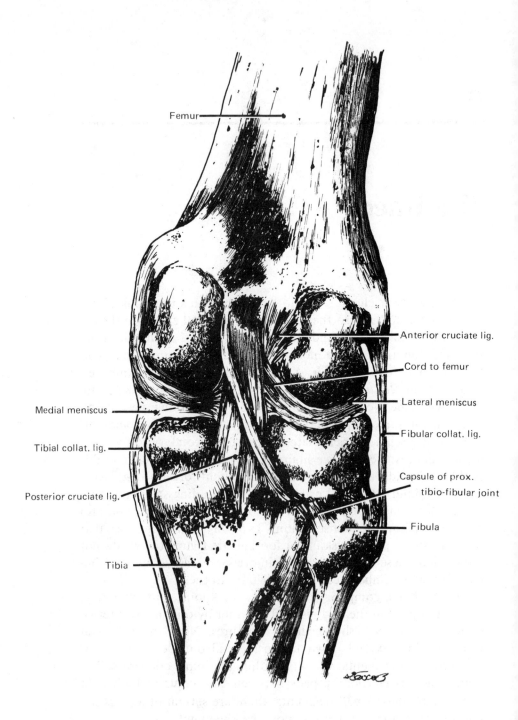

Femur

Anterior cruciate lig.

Cord to femur

Lateral meniscus

Medial meniscus

Fibular collat. lig.

Tibial collat. lig.

Capsule of prox.
tibio-fibular joint

Posterior cruciate lig.

Fibula

Tibia

Fig. 9-1   The Knee (from behind)

The knee gains its strength for accomplishing its crucial function not from the ligaments but from the surrounding muscles. The quadriceps, which are in the front part of the leg, are the most important muscles that affect knee function (Fig. 9-2). As the name implies, there are four individual muscles; they coalesce to form a large tendon that attaches to the upper portion of the tibia. The function of the "quads" is to lift the lower leg on the femur and lock and extend the knee. Also note that the kneecap (patella) is invested within the tendon of the quadriceps muscle. This position improves the muscle's fulcrum, thus allowing for a greater mechanical advantage when the quads function.

The counterpart, or antagonist, to the quadriceps is the hamstring muscles, which are located on the back of the leg, as shown in Fig. 9-3. These muscles flex or unlock the knee. Also important to the knee function are the gastrocnemius muscles; which form the calf muscle. These two muscles originate above the knee and cross it on the way down, forming the Achilles tendon. There are several smaller muscles around the knee that also contribute strength and stability to the joint.

Collectively, the ligaments and muscles function to provide the knee joint with stability and strength. And you cannot underrate the importance of this joint. Consider that at one moment the knee must lock to hold the leg straight (and hence the body upright) and a second later must unlock to provide motion and forward acceleration. This highly "antagonistic" function is one that the knee accomplishes with ease.

Typically, knee pain is caused by a foot, ankle or leg abnormality or from overtraining. This injury is a nagging one at the outset. For instance, a runner, begins to notice a dull, aching pain that comes and goes with activity. Over time this pain may become worse. But there will be no severe pain, unlocking or restriction of motion within the joint. Also, the pain will not be felt deep within the joint; rather, it will be associated with the tendons, ligaments or muscles that surround the joint. The pain appears during or right after activity, but it will not hamper normal walking. We will discuss injuries to the front, back and sides of the knee.

INJURIES TO THE FRONT OF THE KNEE

The main structures to consider in injuries to the front of the knee are the quadriceps muscles and the kneecap or patella. The

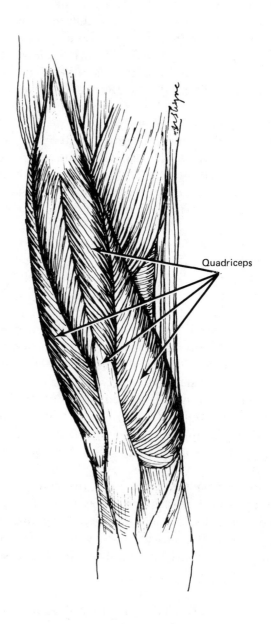

Quadriceps

Fig. 9-2   Anterior Thigh Muscles

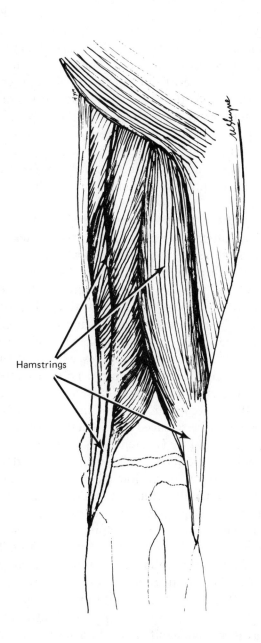

Hamstrings

Fig. 9-3 Posterior Thigh Muscles

most common injury to the front of the knee is chondromalacia patella — the result of cartilage on the undersurface of the knee becoming irritated. This is also known as runner's knee.

Remember, when the foot pronates (turns in), the leg will rotate internally (see Chapter 2). There is an angular relationship between the pull of the quadriceps and the attachment point to the lower leg, as shown in Fig. 9-4a, b. This angle is known as the "Q" angle and any increase of more than 15 degrees is considered abnormal. Remember that the kneecap is inside of the quadriceps tendon and the tendon in turn attaches to the upper portion of the leg. Normally, when the knee is extended from a flexed position, the kneecap is pulled by the quadriceps as the leg assumes a locked position. Try this: sit down and flex and extend your knee. Watch the kneecap or hold your hand on it and feel it move up and down.

There is a deep groove on the front of the femur, in which the kneecap tracks. In order to provide for smooth tracking of the patella, the undersurface of the kneecap as well as the groove on the femur is lined with cartilage, a smooth, glistening, white, oily tissue that allows for smooth motion. Increase the "Q" angle beyond a normal range for the patella and it is pulled off to one side of the groove. This shifting, which occurs with internal rotation, pulls the kneecap to the outside of the groove on the femur. With time and wear these abnormal forces will cause the undersurface of the kneecap to articulate on raw bone. This rubbing on bone causes discomfort. A permanent erosion of cartilage on the undersurface of the kneecap can occur if the problem is not corrected. Cartilage cannot be replaced and surgery is usually required to repair the defect. Disability is often permanent.

What we have just described is chondromalacia patella. However, most active people with a biomechanical problem, such as overpronation, will experience the less severe prechondromalacia patella. Erosion of cartilage has not occurred and knee pain is noticed as a dull ache under or more commonly on the inside or outside of the knee, depending on the foot abnormality. Typically the pain is noticeable only while the person performs his or her sport, or right after. Discomfort increases in severity with an increase in activity. A layoff from activity only temporarily eliminates pain, which reoccurs upon resumption of activity. If a person's activity has increased significantly in a short time, no doubt the knee pain is the result of overuse; rest is essential. If, however, the pain is consistent during exercise and does not clear up over

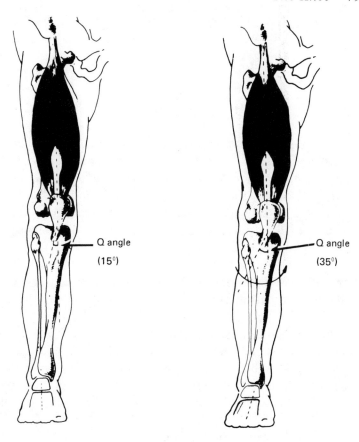

Fig. 9-4a   **Fig. 9-4b**

time, professional help should be sought. We suggest seeing a sports-medicine podiatrist for the typical runner's-type knee.

Treatment of prechondromalacia has two goals. First, the acute phase of the injury receives local physical therapy, such as moist heat and ice, medications, mechanical support such as Ace band-ages or a combination of all of these. Second, it is essential to find the cause of the problem; e.g., overpronation, oversupination, limb length difference. Once we have determined the biomechani-cal problem, we choose a plan of action to correct it. Severe cases often require orthotics. Using proper shoe gear and common sense in training, however, will usually eliminate the minor ailments.

Knee injuries, particularly prechondromalacia, take their time going away. You'll have to live with the frustration of a knee injury that sometimes lingers for several weeks or months. With proper treatment, however, knee pain should gradually disappear, even as activity is increased.

INJURIES TO THE BACK OF THE KNEE

The most common injuries occurring to the back of the knee are related to hamstring tendinitis. The pain is noticeably more sharp than that of other knee injuries. If you suspect a hamstring injury, sit down, relax your leg and feel around the back of the inside and outside of the knee. The hamstring tendons are quite obvious to the touch. If there is any pain along these tendons, then you know you have a hamstring injury.

Hamstring injuries are usually more difficult to treat than other knee injuries. Treatment calls for rest, ice, heat, physical therapy and a determination of the cause. Most hamstring injuries are caused by a biomechanical imbalance. In almost all sports the quadriceps muscles are used more than the hamstrings, and thus are stronger than the hamstrings. So the weaker hamstring tendons are naturally more vulnerable to tearing or pulling at their insertion at the back of the knee. To reduce this imbalance, the hamstring muscles must be strengthened. They should also be stretched prior to any activity.

Pain in the center of the back of the knee is usually associated with a pull of the gastrocnemius muscles. The "gastrocs" consist of two individual muscles arising from behind the knee and coming together at the heel to form the Achilles tendon. Although an injury to the gastrocs is uncommon, it can occur when the Achilles tendon and gastrocs muscles are tight. Many athletes have tight gastrocs. Treatment calls for rest at first; after activity is resumed, stretching the calf muscles is suggested.

INJURIES TO THE SIDE OF THE KNEE

The iliotibial band, shown in Fig. 9-5, runs down the outside of the leg. It originates at the hip and fans out to attach directly below the outside of the knee. Its function is to stabilize the outside of the knee; it is a very large muscle and tendon. Injury to the iliotibial tendon is the most common injury to the outside of the knee joint and is known as an iliotibial band syndrome.

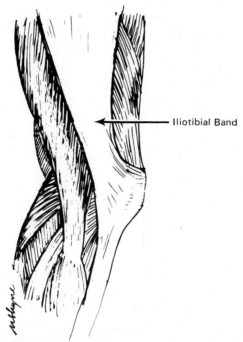

Fig. 9-5 Lateral Thigh Muscles

Any abnormality within the foot or leg can cause the leg to rotate excessively. In a pronated foot, for example, the leg will rotate internally. The iliotibial band, during pronation, is strained as it attempts to pull the leg back into a straight, forward position. This action when repeated time and again can cause an undue stress on the band, particularly at its insertion at the knee. Resulting pain is a dull ache that gets worse with increased activity. Hill workouts, as is true with most knee injuries, tend to make the pain worse.

If you suspect you have an iliotibial band syndrome, palpate the area where the band attaches on the outside of the knee. If you feel any tenderness or pain here, your suspicions will be confirmed.

Injury to the collateral ligaments can also occur. This pain tends to appear suddenly, unlike an iliotibial band pain. It is a distinct, sharp pain. Moreover, the pain tends to be felt deeper within the knee and is well localized to the area of these ligaments. Collateral ligament injuries are not to be treated lightly and immediate treatment should be sought. If left untreated, ligament tears can lead to permanent instability within the knee and chronic pain. Author Harry Hlavac, D.P.M., has this to say about knee injuries in *The Foot Book:* "In the treatment of all overuse injuries, it is very important to consider the causative factor or factors and base your treatment regimen along these lines. Be patient with your treatment plan; results are sometimes slow. But consider any reduction of pain as a step in the right direction. Seek professional care when your condition does not respond to self-treatment. The longer you neglect treatment, the harder it is to reverse the injury process."

PREVENTION OF KNEE INJURIES

Perhaps the most important point in discussing knee injuries is how to prevent them. An athlete's training program calls for common sense to avoid injury. Training, the process of breaking down the body and building it back up to a more efficient level, must be done gradually. Overuse injuries to the knee, and other structures, occur when gradual is forsaken for intense.

One of the best ways to reduce knee injury is to strengthen the muscles that cross this joint. The muscles provide stability to this basically weak joint. Bicycling is one activity that will strengthen muscles around the knee. Also, stretch these muscles prior to activity. Several minutes of stretching prior to activity reduces injuries.

Don't treat knee injuries lightly. As soon as you notice a pain or ache in the knee, stop your activity and determine why it has occurred.

10

Hip and Back Injuries

Foot function has a proven role in causing injuries to the hip and back. All hip and back injuries, however, are not caused by foot imbalances. Many problems here are caused by such factors as disk degeneration or direct trauma. But, conversely, there are many other activity-related injuries to the back and hip that are caused by overuse, secondary to foot and leg imbalances.

HIP INJURIES

Hip injuries are uncommon. The hip, unlike other joints — such as the knee or ankle — rotates in all directions. This ball-and-socket joint is well-designed to take up the stresses generated by the feet and legs.

Hip injuries we do see are often identified as follows: the patient feels a snapping sensation as he moves the hip in a certain position. The "snap" is usually the result of a tendon around the joint popping over a high point on the leg bone. This usually is a painless nuisance. Over time the patient will get used to this "snapping hip." Treatment should be sought, however, if the snapping is associated with pain.

There are many cushioning "pads" built in and around the hip. These pads, called bursae, are the shock absorbers of nearby muscles and tendons that move the hip. Occasionally overuse can cause one of these bursae to become inflamed or irritated, resulting in a bursitis or an inflamed bursae. Treatment is aimed at determining the reason for injury and then instituting local physical therapy. An anti-inflammatory medication is prescribed if the pain is severe. If the bursitis persists, an injection of cortisone to the area is often administered.

Muscle strain and tendinitis can also occur in and around the hip. If this happens, rest and physical therapy are essential. Seek professional help if a hip pain persists. Hip injuries are not to be treated lightly.

BACK INJURIES

We are not implying that the foot is the culprit in causing all back problems. If you have a nagging back pain, get professional help from either a podiatrist, orthopedic surgeon, neurologist, or chiropractor.

We see many active people who have back problems caused by foot imbalances. Abnormal foot function can place stress on the leg, knee, hip and back. Often the back shows the first signs of this increased stress as a dull ache associated with activity. In other words, if you are a runner and your back aches after a run, you should have your feet checked. Again, we want to stress that not all back problems are caused by abnormally functioning feet.

THE BASICS

The human back is composed of thirty-three individual bones called vertebrae. Each vertebra is separated from its neighbor — above and below — by a tough, fibrous cushioning pad called a disk. Fig. 10-1 shows these bones and their supporting disks. The disks serve as shock absorbers and allow the back its great flexibility. Coursing through the center of each vertebra is the spinal cord. The back bones, in addition to being the central pillars of the body, also provide protection for the spinal cord. The spinal cord is a bundle of nerves eminating from the brain and serving as a conduit for sending and receiving messages from the organs and muscles of the body.

As the spinal cord courses down the back, it sends out so-called nerve "roots" between each vertebra (see Fig. 10-2). These roots

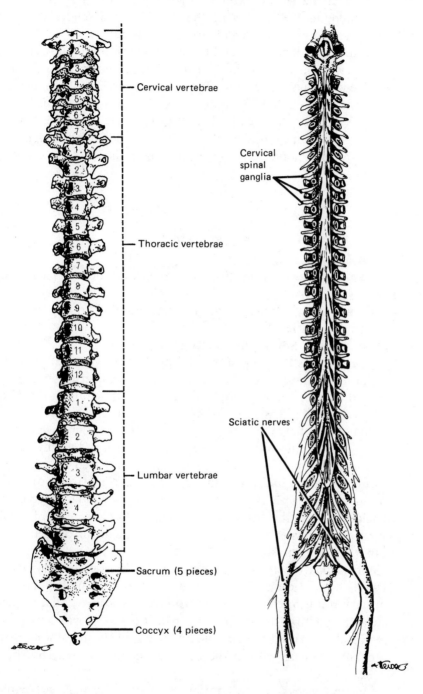

Cervical vertebrae

Thoracic vertebrae

Lumbar vertebrae

Sacrum (5 pieces)

Coccyx (4 pieces)

Cervical
spinal
ganglia

Sciatic nerves

**Fig. 10-1 The Vertebral
Column.** (after Grant's)

**Fig. 10-2 The Spinal
Ganglia.**

function at the level at which they emerge. For instance, a nerve root emerging at the level of the shoulder will send and receive messages from the area in and around the shoulder.

Because the spinal cord and the vertebrae end in the lower back, another way must be found to supply the lower extremities. This is solved by having several of the lower nerve roots merge and form one large, long nerve that serves the legs; this nerve is known as the sciatic nerve. Fig. 10-2 shows this nerve, the largest in the body, as it courses out of the back into the lower extremities. Injury to this nerve is what plagues thousands of active people every year.

SCIATICA

The following conversation was overheard between two runners:

"Charlie. Why'd you stop running last month?"

"I've got sciatica."

"What's that. Sounds like a city in New York."

"Frankly, it's the biggest pain in the ass I've ever encountered."

Among runners, this is hardly an unusual conversation. Almost two out of three active people will, at some time during their life, suffer from sciatica. Sciatica is, literally, a pain in the butt.

The sciatic nerve originates at each side of the lower back, winding down the buttock, the back of the leg and all the way to the foot. Any pull or strain on this nerve will lead to sciatica, a painful and beguiling problem. And to make matters worse, the very nature of activity tends to make the individual more prone to sciatica. With the fitness boom, sciatica has become a big problem. The following is but one of many patient histories that describes the ailment.

Marilyn had been running for six years, averaging forty-five to fifty miles per week. Two months after completing her most recent marathon, she began being troubled by a low-grade, nagging backache. At first she ignored the pain because it was only a nuisance and attributed the discomfort to her recent marathon effort. After all, she had pains in the past that had gone away by themselves.

For two weeks as she continued to run, the pain got worse. Moreover, the pain in her lower back was now beginning to radiate down her right buttock. Concerned about this, she stopped running for one week. During this rest the pain subsided and disappeared completely. So she thought. As soon as she began running it was back. Even more distressing, the pain was radiating down the back of her entire leg and was noticeable not only while running but during the rest of the day. She was unable to run without severe pain; after several more weeks with no improvement, she sought medical help. Our diagnosis — sciatica.

Any irritation to the sciatic nerve, as it leaves the back or along its course down the leg, is called sciatica. There are many causes for this syndrome, but only a few will be discussed here.

Sciatica may be initiated by some antecedent trauma, such as lifting a heavy object while bent over. The nerve is pinched where it leaves the spinal cord. At the moment of injury the pain may be quite severe or it might be mild initially only to become progressively worse. A radiating pain may occur several days or weeks later.

Some people suffer from sciatica as a result of degeneration of the disks. This allows the bony vertebrae to pinch the nerve root as it leaves the spinal cord. Sciatica of this origin is more common in the elderly, where the aging process can cause disk degeneration. Tumors of the lower back can also cause sciatica, but this is rare.

In the active person, however, sciatica tends to occur for different reasons than mentioned above. With running, it is from the constant pounding the body takes. Two to three times a person's body weight is transmitted through each foot and leg at each step during running. For instance, the average runner's feet will strike the ground one thousand times during each mile. Therefore, in a one hundred fifty pound runner, running a ten-kilometer race, the lower extremities must contend with two hundred seventy-nine tons of force. This is obviously a great deal of stress that the body must deal with. The majority of this force is transmitted through the foot, to the leg and eventually the back.

A structural abnormality in the lower extremity will cause this tremendous force, which the body is normally able to contend with, to create any number of problems ranging from foot, ankle, knee, hip and lower back injuries. Abnormalities such as flat feet, high arches, knee problems, and limb length differences are potentially debilitating for the active person. The constant jarring motions of sport accompanied by one of these structural abnormalities can lead to an irritated sciatic nerve.

SYMPTOMS OF SCIATICA

The active person usually first notices sciatica as a subtle, minor ache. There will be a dull, aching pain in the lower back, buttock or thigh. This pain may come after a particularly long or hard workout or race. The pain may subside after several hours only to return once activity is resumed. Resting for a few days will eliminate the pain, but when activity is resumed, the pain reappears. Typically, the pain is not severe enough to limit activity. But over several days or weeks, the pain intensifies. Moreover, depending on the type of problem, the pain will begin to radiate deep in the buttocks, on one side, and eventually down the back of the leg. At this point, the pain is usually enough to cause the person to cease all activity. Rest tends to alleviate the symptoms but, unlike at the outset, the pain never completely disappears and is present at all hours of the day. The pain increases when doing straight-leg raises, curving the spine, sneezing or even coughing. These activities place additional stress on the already irritated nerve.

The lower-back pain may soon disappear, although pain remains in the buttock and/or back of the leg. Pressing on the back of the leg brings severe pain. What we have described is a classic case of sciatica. It can, in extreme cases, make walking impossible.

This example is an extreme case. The "average" sciatica is less severe. Typically, a runner can jog a short distance before the pain becomes too intense. Sciatica pain causes a burning sensation; the affected limb may feel like it's going numb. With time, the individual changes his stride while walking and running in order to compensate for and alleviate the sciatic pain. In other words, if a person has pain in the right leg, his tendency will be to favor the left leg. Secondary problems may occur as a result of this — tendinitis, knee pain or even stress fractures.

The secondary problem may be the reason for a person eventually seeking medical help. That's why it is imperative that an examination reveal the true cause of the injury. For example, if an individual comes in with a stress fracture, the root of the problem might be his overcompensating for back pain. The overcompensation placed undue stress on the foot. In addition to treating the stress fracture, the sciatica must be remedied.

DIAGNOSIS

A complete medical history is taken before making a diagnosis, which will rule out disk degeneration, herniation or tumors of the spine where the symptoms of sciatica are present. Most healthy people suffering from sciatica do not have these ailments. And the pain in these cases tends to be quite different from that of an active person who has sciatica.

In gathering information for a diagnosis, we ask the patient when the pain started, what self-treatment was done — if any — what type of exercise he pursues, when the pain occurs, if the pain has gotten worse, what other pains have occurred, and so on. A physical exam is then given; we try to reproduce the symptoms and find out if there are any structural problems with his back, legs, knees or feet.

Now I'll explain why a foot imbalance can cause sciatica and back problems. As you will recall from earlier reading, at each step the heel moves from a position of being turned in (supinated) to one of being turned out (pronated) and back again. Heel movement is essential for proper foot function. An extreme amount of force is generated at each step in sports and for this force to be rendered harmless it must be controlled and dissipated evenly. If it is not controlled, injury can occur in the foot, ankle, knee, hip, lower back and to the sciatic nerve.

In addition to an overpronated foot placing undue stress on the leg and back, there is a secondary problem that furthers your vulnerability to sciatic nerve injury. When the foot pronates, the leg tends to rotate internally.

The kneecaps (which reflect the position of the entire leg in this case) will be pointing in instead of straight ahead. This internal rotation of the leg will cause the front part of the pelvis to drop slightly forward, a technically complex maneuver. The result of this tilting is that the sciatic nerve, which runs through the back of the leg, is stretched. This stretching, in addition to the tremendous force being placed on the legs by the abnormal foot function, can cause sciatica.

Other imbalances can cause sciatica, like a leg length difference. The longer leg takes more pounding. Also, the foot of the longer leg usually pronates excessively in order to functionally shorten the leg. This can lead to sciatica on the long leg.

Another problem afflicting some people is a high-arch foot. Although less common than a flat foot, the high-arch foot is less able to absorb shock than either flat or regular feet. A foot that is unable to absorb shock can lead to sciatic nerve irritation.

Lumbar lordosis, or sway back, can also lead to sciatica. The lordosis spine is excessively curved, which causes the sciatic nerve to stretch. Lordosis can be congenital. However, any activity that strengthens back muscles can lead to an acquired lordosis, causing sciatica.

Sciatica should not be treated lightly. A sciatic nerve can be permanently injured, leading to muscle wasting in the leg and foot. The injury may eventually require surgery.

TREATMENT

Treatment of sciatica is twofold: 1) to eliminate the acute symptoms (i.e.: the pain) and 2) to determine its origin. Reducing the nerve inflammation will eliminate the pain. Rest is essential. Unlike some injuries where activity may be continued at a reduced level while healing, back injuries require rest — from several days to weeks. By rest we don't mean being bedridden, but rather a complete cessation of any activity that might irritate the nerve.

Rest is also important in determining the seriousness of the injury. For example, if after a week of rest the pain is still bad, we know the injury is severe; the treatment plan is altered to accommodate this.

Moist heat over the affected area will reduce inflammation and speed recovery. Although we are not advocates of "a pill for every problem," anti-inflammatory medications have a definite role in the treatment of the more severe cases of sciatica. We prescribe a short-term course of non-cortisone, anti-inflammatory medication for five to seven days, followed by a consistent dosage of aspirin, if necessary.

Once the severe pain is brought under control, which may take from hours to several days, we have the patient begin a stretching and strengthening program. This is done to correct the existing muscular imbalances, which caused the sciatica.

As we initiate this short-term treatment we also begin working on the root cause. If, for example, we can show through a careful history and physical examination that the patient's sciatica is caused by a limb length difference, then we construct a heel lift for the short side. Similarly, if we attribute sciatica to a flat foot, we construct an orthotic to correct this problem. We have found orthotics to be extremely effective in solving a majority of problems associated with sciatica and lower-back problems. Even a mild foot imbalance associated with sciatica is benefited by orthotics.

PREVENTION

More important than treatment of sciatica injury is its prevention. What can be done to prevent the injury from occurring? When dealing with back injuries, the old adage, "An ounce of prevention is worth a pound of cure," certainly holds true. That means stretching and strengthening the lower back muscles, which will increase the flexibility of the spine.

Know how to lift heavy objects. Improper lifting can strain the back. The proper way to pick up a heavy object is to keep your back *straight*, bend your legs at the knees, and lift with your legs, *not* your back. Remember: bend your legs and lift with your legs.

Pain is the body's warning sign of an impending problem, and this pain should not be ignored. This is particularly true for back injuries; a mild back pain can lead to a very serious, debilitating injury.

There are many causes of back pain. Is it just overuse? Is there a structural problem like flat feet, high-arch feet, or a limb length difference? Is there an old injury? Is there stress on your job? Are you sleeping on the wrong kind of mattress? These are potential causes for back and sciatica problems.

11

Self-Treatment

Self-treatment begins with prevention. Thorough understanding of your body, your sport and its equipment is instrumental in preventing injury in any exercise program.

The first building block of prevention is the warmup. This calls for slow, relaxed movements similar to those of your sport. Avoid high-speed movements or ballistic stretching until you are thoroughly warmed up. Start slowly and gradually increase your tempo. Many healthy runners I know will jog slowly for about a mile and then begin a slow muscle stretching program for ten to fifteen minutes. After that they go on their run. When you are through with your exercise, warm down slowly and don't allow your muscles to get chilled. Make sure you put on a sweat suit or otherwise stay warm after exercise. Continue walking to prevent the muscles from tightening; this also allows your blood pressure to decrease gradually. If you are going to resume activity some time after cooling down, then warm up again slowly.

Know which muscles are going to be involved in your sport and which ones may be along for the ride. Do not ignore the ride-along muscles or you'll wind up with imbalances. If you are a runner, this means strengthening your hamstring muscles and upper body.

Has it been quite a few years since you last exercised; say *ten* years or more? Then keep repeating to yourself that you are unconditioned and that it is going to take a while to get in shape. That fifty-two second quarter mile you did in high school may be more like a two-minute quarter mile twenty years later.

Get good equipment. We can't stress enough the necessity for good equipment, especially shoes if you are a runner. Running shoes can make or break an athlete (See Chapter 14).

MDFS

This acronymn, originally described by Dr. Lowell Weil, D.P.M., refers to mechanical, drugs, flexibility and strength. This is the approach we use in treatment of an injury. All of the components of MDFS include RICE. We will explain the components of MDFS here.

MECHANICAL

Rest. Something all of us should do from time to time. But when you are training for a specific goal and get injured, rest is the last thing you'll want to do. Or should. For every week of rest you lose approximately two to three weeks of training. Here's how to get around the dilemma. Rest the injury and pursue other physical activities to keep up your aerobic, cardiovascular, and muscular endurance. For example, if you have a heel bruise from running, you can always bicycle, swim, lift weights, or run in a swimming pool until the heel injury disappears. Keep in mind that most overuse injuries take six weeks to heal. Although you can probably resume your main activity much sooner than that, it must be at a reduced level. You may have discomfort in the area of the injury that goes away after a mile of running. If so, you may continue running without fear of reinjury. If the pain persists after a mile or two or gets worse, discontinue the activity. You need more rest.

Compression. Compression is valuable with soft-tissue injuries, especially those accompanied with swelling. Compression can take many forms, utilizing Ace bandages, Elastoplast tape, unna boot, which is a zinc-oxide-impregnated gauze wrapping, and other materials. Compression prevents fluid from accumulating in the tissue spaces, which causes immobility and pain. If you have an acute injury such as a sprain, immediately apply compression to keep the swelling down. With a long-standing, chronic problem such as a tendinitis or a muscle strain, compression will keep the area from swelling and provide support. An Ace bandage works well because it is easily applied and removed. Always remember to apply it snugly, starting away from the body, such as on the front part of the foot. Loosen it as you get closer to the body, such as toward the ankle. This technique provides a milking effect when ambulating. Elastoplast tape can be purchased in a drug store and used in combination with a zinc-oxide wrap or unna boot. This will make what is known as a soft cast. If you feel numbness or pain, loosen the compression dressing and reapply it less tightly.

Elevation. Elevation is utilized with rest and compression. The injured area should be kept at least at heart level. Elevation promotes drainage, which reduces swelling. This allows the tissues to heal more quickly.

Aperature pads. We mentioned these in the discussion of corns and calluses. There are many different types and sizes on the market, but their purpose is the same: to accommodate the injured area. Sometimes the pad is not thick enough and/or is easily compressed. The minimum thickness we use is one-eighth inch (felt), the thickest generally one-half inch. Felt can be bought with adhesive on one side, thereby eliminating the need for taping. If you have an opening in the skin from a severe blister or an infected corn or callus, always fill the aperature pad with a topical antibiotic; cotton should cover it, if it will not create discomfort; then apply tape to hold the aperature pad in place. This will reduce the chance of infection.

Taping. Taping provides support, compression, and immobilization of the injured area. There are as many different ways of applying tape as there are trainers. Before applying tape, find out if you are allergic to adhesive, and if you're going to apply tape regularly use Pre-wrap or J-wrap — a thin, cushioning material that prevents the tape from irritating the skin.

A very common method of taping is known as the low-dye strap. We use this more often than any other method. Here is how it's done: First, you will need seven strips — three to go around the back of the heel and four to go underneath the foot. The purpose of this taping is to hold up the medial or inside part of the foot; it will help relieve problems such as posterior tibial tendinitis, plantar fasciitis, and heel spur pain. Fig. 11-1a shows how to measure the length of the three straps going around the back of the heel. These will run from approximately the outside mid-foot to the inside mid-foot. The next four pieces of tape will run from the outside ankle bone to the inside ankle bone, underneath the foot. Fig. 11-1b shows the first tape as it is applied, starting from the outside, going around the heel to the inside of the foot; keep the foot pointed down and inward at all times while the tape is

Low- Dye Wrap

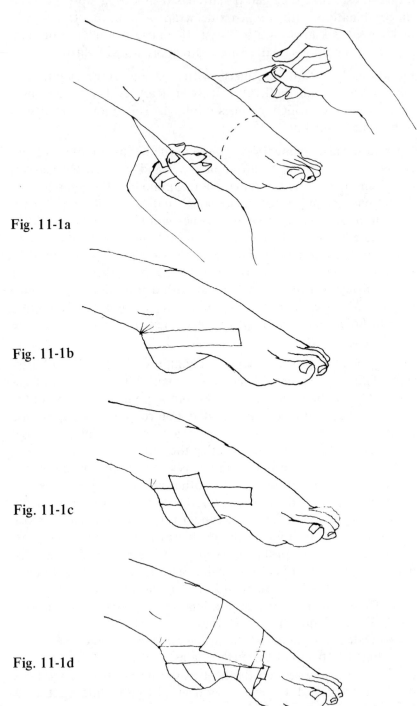

Fig. 11-1a

Fig. 11-1b

Fig. 11-1c

Fig. 11-1d

being applied. Fig. 11-1c shows the second tape being applied from the outside ankle area underneath the heel to the inside ankle area. The application of strips is then alternated from behind the heel to underneath the foot. Fig. 11-1d shows the final application. This low-dye strap will temporarily eliminate many problems of over-pronation.

Heel lifts. Heel lifts can be utilized for many problems, such as Achilles tendinitis, plantar fasciitis, retro calcaneal exostosis, and others. Heel lifts should be made of thick, non-compressible material. A heel lift should be at least one-half inch thick. Cork or a hard shoe padding felt in quarter-inch thicknesses are preferred because they are easily adjustable for more or less thickness. When you stop utilizing the heel lift you may have to begin a stretching program to lengthen the calf muscle, especially if you have been wearing the lift for a long time. Make sure you cut the lift to conform to the heel of your shoes; carry it no farther forward than about three inches inside your shoe from the heel. Taper the front edge for a comfortable fit.

Wedges. Wedges are a poor man's orthotic. They fit under the heel and reduce pronation, hopefully enough to clear up a syndrome of overpronation. We use half-inch hard felt and a skiving knife to create a wedge with the thickest part on the back, inside edge, tapering off to the front, outside edge. The wedge also tapers toward the front part of the foot and the outside, back heel. The corners are rounded to fit the heel counter, and the wedge should extend no farther forward than the heel of the foot. The thickest part always goes under the back, inside edge of the heel. The wedges will comform to your heel, but compress with time.

DRUGS

The term is used loosely here to include ice, heat, and some over-the-counter anti-inflammatory medications. Certain drugs used with discretion can be of value in reducing inflammation and speed healing.

Ice. Ice can almost never be overused, but there are appropriate times when it should be applied. Ice is most effective within the first twenty-four hours of an injury. If there is considerable swelling, place cracked ice in a plastic bag and apply it on top of a washcloth that covers the injury. The washcloth will prevent frostbite. With more acute injuries, ice is most effective when applied

in the first twenty-four to forth-eighty hours. If there is considerable swelling, you can alternate heat application with ice to create
a milking effect, which will be discussed further in the section on
heat.

Ice massage is highly recommended for an overuse injury such
as a tendinitis, and should be done after running. We like to freeze
water in a paper cup. Then peel the top of the cup off to expose
the ice and move the ice in circles over the injured area. The ice
will sting, numb and then cause redness. The redness is the result
of capillaries dilating from constriction. Metabolites build up when
capillaries are constricted, and dilation occurs. This creates a blood
flushing effect and helps reduce swelling. Ice massage should last
for about ten to fifteen minutes; a ten-minute ice massage is the
equivalent of a forty-five minute ice pack application. Ice massage
beyond fifteen minutes is not beneficial; you may get frostbite.

What do you use before an activity, ice or heat? This is still an
issue of controversy. Although ice does provide a desired flushing
effect as does heat, it has been our experience that applying heat
to an injury prior to exercising and using ice after activity is the
best regimen. But if applying heat prior to exercise creates swelling
in the problem area, ice would be the treatment of choice.

Heat. Heat can be applied in the form of hot towels, lamps, heat-
ers, electric pads, ointments, hot baths, and so on. For generalized
aching after some strenuous activity, nothing feels better or is better than a hot bath or Jacuzzi. For isolated pains like tendinitis,
we recommend a hydroculator or a steam pack for self-treatment.
These can be purchased at most medical equipment stores.

Generally, for an injury that is more than forth-eight hours old,
chronic, or non-swelling, a steam pack is suggested. Make sure you
wrap enough layers of towel around the steam pack, commonly
four to six; use it a minimum of three times per day, usually twenty
minutes each time, and prior to activity. You can save time by
using two or three steam packs at once, if necessary. A steam pack
has a vasodilating effect, loosens tight muscles for extra flexibility
and feels good. Be careful not to burn your skin, and store the
steam pack in the freezer to prevent mildew.

A heating pad provides mainly cutaneous or skin surface heat
and does not get deep into the tissues, as does a steam pack.
Creams such as Ben Gay and Atomic Balm are nothing more than
skin irritants; blood flows to the area of application to remove the
irritant, at which time blood circulates through the sore tissues.
They work quite well and should be applied prior to an activity,

after the steam pack has been used. First allow the skin to cool. If the cream is applied to warm skin with open pores, considerable stinging can result.

Aspirin. Over-the-counter anti-inflammatory medications such as aspirin are effective (see Chapter 16). Aspirin should be used in lieu of non-aspirin, pain-relieving products such as Tylenol or Datril. These are not anti-inflammatory. Aspirin can be more effective if you take it about twenty minutes prior to using a steam pack. Then, when the steam pack is applied the aspirin is already circulating in your blood and more of it will be drawn to the injury by the dilation from the steam pack. If aspirin tends to upset your stomach, try a buffered aspirin such as Bufferin or Ascriptin. Aspirin will cause some blood loss in the stomach, so it should not be used in excess. There are many other potential side effects, which should be taken as signs for immediate cessation of the medication. Also, taking two aspirin prior to activity will help reduce pain, though not so much as to mask the injury and cause further damage.

FLEXIBILITY

Do you wake up in the morning, roll out of bed, decide to do some stretching exercises, bend over and discover you can't touch your knees? If that's true, my friend, it is time to begin a serious stretching program. Unfortunately, this probably sounds like most of us to a certain degree, especially if you have been into long-distance running for quite some time. We know of only one person who stretches enough, and that is Jean Couch, author of *Runner's World Yoga Book*.

Proper flexibility is a must for injury prevention and treatment. We can't tell you how many people we've seen with pulled hamstrings, calf muscles, and sore Achilles tendons, all of which could have been avoided with a good stretching program. Some years ago a study was done at the Honolulu Marathon, which showed that more runners who stretch tend to get injured than those who do not stretch. Unfortunately, this caused many people to stop stretching. We firmly believe that the people who did get injured from stretching were doing it improperly and thereby increasing the risk of injury.

Many times before a road race you will see contestants near the course bouncing up and down trying to touch their toes. They think that this ballistic bouncing is stretching their muscles.

Nothing could be further from the truth. Ballistic stretches such as the ones just mentioned further shorten the muscles. The muscles contract to protect themselves from injury. Because muscles have a shorter length at rest — the result of repetitive contraction and ballistic stretching — it is imperative that stretching be done properly.

When you go into stretch, extend to the point where you begin to feel the stretching sensation, then relax the stretch a bit, and hold it for a minimum of thirty seconds. You should never feel discomfort or pain. If you do, you're causing microscopic tears in the connective tissue. If you go on to other stretches and return later to the one you started with, you will notice that you can comfortably stretch a little farther. Extend until you can feel the stretch, back off a little, and then hold it for a minimum of thirty seconds.

When an injury has healed enough to allow stretching, a good procedure is to apply a steam pack to the injured muscle, stretch, and stay stretched for up to an hour. Before removing the heat and letting up on the stretch, apply an ice pack to the area that was just heated. Cooling the stretched muscle allows it to remain in a stretched position, i.e., the length at rest is greater. The benefit from this treatment was recently published in the magazine *Physician and Sports Medicine*. In fact, the article points out that muscle injuries subjected to temperatures of 102 to 110 degrees Fahrenheit and held at those temperatures for twenty to sixty minutes, then cooled down for ten minutes while held in the stretched position, showed quicker healing than other methods of treatment. When you finish your workout you should do some more stretching before hitting the shower.

Someone once likened stretching cold muscles to trying to bend a dry sponge. A wet sponge is easily bent, much as a muscle that has been filled with blood. Think of your muscles as having the flexibility of a dry sponge when you start your activities. A slow warmup and some pre-exercise stretching will "soak" the muscles and make them limber. It is also advisable to stretch in the morning; your muscles will have a longer resting length during the day and stretch out more quickly for your afternoon or evening workout. Morning stretching routines demand extra caution; the muscles are not profused with blood as they would be at the end of the day or after activity. For more on stretching, check with your local YMCA, read a book on the subject or take a yoga or stretching class. After a short while, you should be able to roll out of bed and touch those knees, perhaps even the toes.

STRENGTH

Strengthening the injured muscles should begin as soon as most of their normal range of motion returns. Invariably, you will lose some muscle strength because of the enforced layoff. Do *not* begin strengthening too soon; you can easily reinjure yourself. This often happens when people return to a sport from which they haven't fully recovered, especially in terms of strength. There are many different methods for strengthening an injured part, four of which will be discussed here.

Isometrics. Isometrics is the first type of strength exercise that you should do following an injury. This consists of contracting or flexing your muscles around the injured area. Restrict all other body movement. This exercise can be done any place at any time and with a minimal risk of injury. Your first isometrics workout should last about five or ten minutes; contract, relax, contract, relax. Follow this with range of motion or flexibility exercises. Soreness is not unusual after such a workout, especially if your layoff has been a long one.

Resistance. Resistance exercises follow isometrics, but only when isometrics can be done without discomfort. Constant resistance is the movement of weight against gravity — a barbell, dumbbell, a purse filled with sand. Start this exercise by using just the weight of your body, such as lifting your leg, bending your ankle up and down, or straightening your leg out at the knee. As this becomes easier, you can begin to use more weight. If you have a leg or foot injury, weighted boots or ankle weights are helpful. Your local health club will have a full line of weight machines, or you can buy a barbell weight set for home use.

Variable resistance. This requires expensive equipment; few people can afford to buy a machine, such as that made by Nautilus or Universal, for home use. These machines provide uniform resistance during the entire range of motion in the exercise. Muscle endurance as well as muscle strength is increased. There are machines for specific muscle groups.

Isokinetics. Also known as constant speed exercise, isokinetics is done utilizing a machine similar to a Cybex or Orthotron. These machines provide constant speed instead of constant resistance. The harder you push against the machine the more resistance you feel. So, the force exerted while the muscle shortens is at its maximum level. The Cybex machine is quite useful in determining strength percentage differences between muscle groups. For instance, in long-distance running, the quadriceps muscles will become considerably stronger than the hamstrings, thereby making the hamstrings susceptible to strain and/or rupture. Utilizing a Cybex machine, the percentage strength difference can be found, and if the quadriceps are more than 40 percent stronger than the hamstrings, a strengthening program is essential for the hamstrings.

Prior to an exercise session you should always warm up the muscle or muscles involved. This can be done with steam packs or gentle range-of-motion exercises. If you still have some swelling from the injury, ice is recommended prior to the session, and ice is always recommended after an exercise session. Continue your strengthening program until recovery is complete.

12

A Visit to the Podiatrist

You have read all about your problem, tried self-treatment, and you still are not getting any better. Now what? First, ask your friends if they or anyone they know have had a similar problem. If they went to a podiatrist, was he involved in the particular sport in which the injury occurred? A doctor familiar with sportsmedicine who has previously treated a similar injury is one step ahead of the game.

Once you are sure the doctor is an expert at treating sports-related injuries, give his office a call. Do not hesitate to ask about the cost right away. The cost of an office visit is generally a standard rate, which increases with number of required X-rays, lab tests, orthotics, and so on. There is good reason why the exact fee cannot be given over the phone. While the initial office visit might be $35, X-rays could be an extra $30 or more, depending on how many views the doctor needs.

For the first visit to a podiatrist, you should bring the following: brief, written outline chronicling your problem with time spans from initial onset, to subsequent treatment; the nature of the self-treatment and its affect; the shoes worn in your activity; and, if possible, wear your running shorts or bring them to the office. At the office you will be asked to fill out a medical and personal history form. Take advantage of any free brochures you find in the waiting room. The doctor may refer to them when discussing your problem.

Then you will meet the doctor. He will ask questions regarding your injury and about past injuries. He will give a brief physical exam, usually consisting of testing reflexes, taking your pulse, and a range-of-motion test. You might then be asked to walk or run; the podiatrist calls this a kinetic gait analysis. By watching your gait he can better determine the function of the subtalar joint, observe leg function and movement, and check for bow-leggedness, curvature of the spine and hip mechanics.

After the kinetic gait analysis the doctor might request X-rays to evaluate joint stability and to look for bone abnormalities. The doctor should show you the X-rays and explain what he is looking for, where your problem may lie, and why the problem developed.

Once the tests have been completed, the doctor should be able to give his assessment, and make recommendations for treatment. In our practice we always try the most conservative treatment first. Sometimes the patient has already tried the conservative treatment without success and comes to the office seeking a quick cure. But there is no panacea.

There are, however, treatments available only in a doctor's office that can speed recovery. Those combined with a foot insert and range-of-motion exercises are methods for healing an injury.

Ultrasound

Ultrasound is a powerful heating agent that can be effective even in deep muscle tissue. It is a high-frequency sound wave generated from alternating current that produces a mechanical vibration of eight hundred thousand to one million cycles per second. Ultrasound causes molecular vibrations, which increase temperature.

Ultrasound is effective in treating overuse problems such as bursitis and tendinitis. It can also be used for resorption of adhesions following surgery.

A transducer is placed in contact with the skin, usually through a coupling medium such as water, glycerin, mineral oil, or transmission gel. An intensity control and timer give the ability to use ultrasound on various parts of the body.

Ultrasound improves deep tissue blood flow, thereby relaxing muscles, increasing metabolism and connective tissue extensibility. Ultrasound used in conjunction with deep tissue massage will help break up muscle spasms and further reduce inflammation. Usually the doctor will suggest daily treatments of ultrasound for the first week or two, diminishing to two or three visits thereafter as the problem begins clearing. The doctor may also ask you to utilize a steam pack at home in conjunction with ultrasound treatment, along with ice massage of the area.

Whirlpool

This treatment is utilized to relax muscles and bring blood to the surrounding areas. It is commonly used for a total extremity rather than for a specific muscle. Water temperature is usually 95 to 105 degrees.

Deep Tissue Massage

The doctor or assistant may give a deep tissue massage. Self-treatment is not generally effective, because the patient fails to massage deeply. We will show the patient how it is done, how it should feel, and request that a family member or friend continue with the treatment at home. The person giving the massage should follow instructions closely; if done improperly or too often, it can cause damage.

Range-of-Motion Exercises

In many situations, a doctor, assistant, or physical therapist will perform passive and active range-of-motion exercises, especially post-injury, post-cast, or post-surgery.

Other treatment modalities include surgery, medication and orthotic fitting. These subjects are dealt with in other chapters.

Follow-up visits may or may not be necessary. In most cases, when the problem is minor the doctor will give self-treatment directions and request that you abstain from exercises until the acute phase of the injury has passed. If the problem persists or reoccurs, you should make a return visit. In more severe cases, return visits might be daily, weekly, biweekly.

When you leave the office have all of your questions answered, and be sure you understand your treatment procedure. Write your instructions down so that you do not forget them. But do not hesitate to call the doctor if there is an unanswered question. Keep in mind that this chapter is what we do and our recommendation. You will find many variations on this theme.

13

Sport-Specific Injuries

Sport-specific injuries stem from two major activities: those with exclusively forward movement, such as running, and those with side-to-side movement, such as tennis, soccer, or football. Orthotics, either soft or hard, have proven over the years to have an important place in treating many kinds of sports injuries. Their use will be mentioned in conjunction with sports injuries.

Running and Race Walking

Because these sports are primarily without lateral movement, correcting abnormal foot motion is less difficult. The race walker's risk of injury is reduced further because one foot must constantly be in contact with the ground; body weight impact becomes less of a factor.

Ailments associated with running and race walking include overpronation, plantar fasciitis, posterior tibial tendinitis, runner's knee, and stress fractures. Rigid orthotics are often successful in reducing the incidence of these injuries.

Sprinting and steeplechasing require different orthotics than those used in road running. Since footstrike in sprinting is generally on the ball of the foot, rigid control is not needed; a sport orthotic is prescribed. Steeplechase requires a soft or sport orthotic to prevent its fracture when landing on the top of the steeplechase barrier. Some steeplechase competitors have made the mistake of wearing a rigid orthotic, which shatters or cracks inside the wearer's shoe on making contact with the top of the barrier.

Injuries usually seen in these two events are capsulitis of the metatarsal heads from improper shock absorption or spikes pushing into the bottom of the foot.

Soccer

Next to runners in numbers of patients, we see soccer players. The majority of players are in their early teens so we see a lot of calcaneal apophysitis inflammation of the growth area in the heel. This is usually caused by wearing shoes with spikes underneath the heel. The problem is easily controlled by inserting a heel cup and sport orthotics. In some cases where the foot is extremely pronated, rigid orthotics are prescribed, usually with Spenco or other insole material glued to the top of the orthotic to prevent slippage on the orthotic.

Other injuries common to soccer players are sprained ankles, contusions or bruises, and sore knees. The knee injuries are generally traumatic in origin.

Football

Treatment of football injuries runs the gamut. Football backs and ends, by making quick lateral movements and constantly sprinting, often have tendinitis, sprained ankles, and forefoot problems. A soft orthotic works well.

Linemen, who make few quick movements and face different obstacles than backs, do quite well with plastic orthotics. These provide stability and do not flatten out. Also, backs who have severe overpronation will do well with rigid orthotics.

Baseball

Generally, baseball players do well with rigid orthotics because they need foot control in running. Batting is different from running but a rigid orthotic is still our first choice unless it is not tolerated, in which case sport orthotics would be prescribed. Standing for the length of time players do in the field, we have found the rigid orthotic to be more comfortable.

Injuries associated with baseball include forefoot injuries from the twisting common to batting and sprinting; tendinitis from the running, and bruises from the sliding. We have seen feet, ankles and legs so badly injured from a slide that the players must end their careers.

Tennis

Tennis requires quick movement in all directions. Rigid orthotics do not work well. They reduce mobility and the player may slide on the orthotic as it sits in the shoe bed. Sport orthotics work best.

Problem areas: forefoot, heel, medial leg, blisters and toenails. Bad toenails are what we see the most of in this sport.

Basketball

Sport orthotics, which are more pliable than the plastic version, are prescribed in this sport known for jumping and lateral movement. The rigid orthotic, by eliminating excessive pronation, might even increase the risk of a sprain for those with weak ankles. Taping combined with soft orthotics works well for the player with weak ankles.

Problem areas: forefoot capsulitis, plantar heel bruises, fractured metatarsals caused by a player landing on another's foot, and sprained ankles.

Snow Skiing

Snow skiing has a special place in Dr. Zamzow's heart, not to mention his leg and ankle; it is the sport that introduced him to podiatric medicine. In December 1967, on the last run of the day, (which is when most injuries occur) he went into a side stop, hit some ice, and crashed. His right fibular malleolus was fractured and every muscle in his left leg was torn. Eventually pain developed under the left heel from the posterior tibial muscle being stretched and plantar fasciitis developed. A visit to a podiatrist resulted in orthotics being prescribed and the heel problem cleared up.

Most ski-related foot pains result from improper foot function, unlike the case of Dr. Zamzow, where the skiing caused injury. Recently, orthotics have been used to eliminate the need for cants on skis. The orthotics − by correcting pronation − have also been found to give improved edge control. By correcting a foot pronation with a shoe insert, supination and pronation take place around the neutral position, thus eliminating the need for cants.

Many ski shops have jumped on the band wagon regarding orthotics for their skiers in lieu of cants. But they can do more harm than good without a thorough examination. Also, the appropriate orthotic for the skier might not be utilized. We recommend taking your ski boots to a podiatrist if you are having problems or, if orthotics are prescribed, taking them with you when buying a new pair of ski boots.

Bicycling

We are beginning to see more and more of our runners from years past coming back with injury generated by bicycling. The popularity of the sport as a means of injury-free training is well known. However, occasional problems do occur. Unfortunately, because propulsion is mostly achieved through the ball of the foot, correcting biomechanical irregularities is difficult. Forefoot varus or valgus can be controlled by applying a slight cant to the bike pedal. This will help control the subtalar joint around its neutral position and, it is hoped, eliminate some problems generally associated with the knee.

Ice Skating and Roller Skating

These two sports require considerable ankle motion, especially so with roller skating. Since ice skating hinges on controlling the edge of the blade in relationship to the ice, we are concerned with maintaining the subtalar joint in the neutral position. So rigid orthotics are generally prescribed for ice skaters.

The wheels of the roller skater have to be on the ground, so there tends to be more motion throughout the subtalar joint, generally requiring softer orthotics.

Golf

Golf is somewhat like baseball in biomechanical demands on the feet and legs, although not as strenuous. A twisting motion accompanies the swing of the club, and of course you should walk the course. We usually see patients with metatarsal problems, such as calluses and capsulitis, which result from the swing. Because the swing mechanics take place mostly on the forefoot, rigid orthotics work well. If the rigid orthotics are not tolerated when swinging the golf club, semi-rigid orthotics are prescribed.

Dancing

Each of the many different dance steps has its unique demands on the feet. Aerobic dancing is not immune and we are seeing patients injured because of it. Dance injuries do have certain similarities, however.

Posterior tibial tendinitis, pain in the bottom of the heel, capsulitis, and disco digit are known to aerobic and modern dance. Unfortunately, it is difficult to treat injuries associated with overpronation when women wear fashionable dance shoes.

Ballet involves toe standing, leaps and turns. A ballet dancer cannot wear orthotics while performing, but soft padding has been used successfully.

14

Shoes

Why do we need shoes? Ancient Greek Olympians never wore shoes, and even some current great runners — Bruce Tulloh from England to name one — never wore shoes while racing. Just look outside for your answer. A jungle of concrete and asphalt is quickly carpeting our world. Running on concrete in bare feet is nobody's treat. Add to that, modern-day glass, nails, etc., and shoes become a necessity.

It is impossible to recommend a shoe here because of biomechanical differences between individuals, but we can give basic recommendations that apply to everyone. First, though, an anatomy lesson for a running shoe.

Fig. 14-1 shows a running shoe. The three major portions are the outersole, midsole and the upper.

OUTERSOLE

Two outersole factors are paramount: its carbon compound and the surface area contacting the ground. Therefore, the first part of the outersole to wear out (because of footstrike patterns) is the outside corner of the heel of the outersole. In many shoes this has been strengthened with the addition of more rubber. Also, the more carbon that is added to the rubber of the outersole, the longer it will wear. A good outersole lasts about five hundred

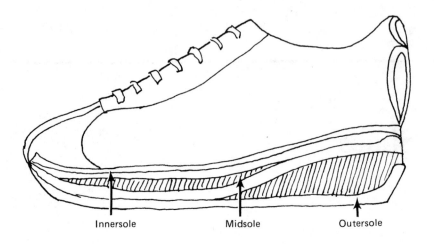

Fig. 14-1 **Cross-Section of a Running Shoe**

miles, although some outersoles are so soft that they barely last through a marathon. If you happen to purchase an otherwise good shoe with a soft outersole, as soon as it wears through to the softer midsole, have it replaced with a high-carbon outersole. Many outersoles, especially at the area of greatest wear, can be rebuilt at home by applying a liquid glue like Shoe Goo. Do not apply so much glue that a higher ridge than the rest of the sole is formed.

MIDSOLE

A midsole provides cushioning and control. The most commonly used midsole material is EVA, or ethyl vinyl acetate. The hardness of this EVA is measured in durometers. The greater the durometer reading, the harder the sole. EVA is a foam rubber permeated by tiny air bubbles or air cells. Some shoes that have a lot of air cells are called "blown" EVA. This is generally found on midsoles that are one color, usually white. On other midsoles you might see two different colors, indicating different durometers — one for cushioning and one for control.

There have been many variations in the scheme of making a better midsole. Some manufacturers have utilized removable plugs that insert at the side of the midsole — color-coded for shock absorption properties — plugs on the bottom of the sole, air channels or bladders, built-in wedges and flared heels that give a spoiler effect to the shoe.

As more and more people began taking to the roads, people who had never been physically active, shoe manufacturers started making shoes with softer, thicker midsoles. They wanted to reduce the footstrike impact to a minimum to reduce the risk of injury. It became a contest to see who could provide the most cushioning. But things got out of hand. One of the most important considerations in shoe design — foot control — was cast aside. The softer the midsoles became, the more injured runners we saw. That there would have to be a reverse in the trend toward cushioning was soon obvious.

Soft-soled shoes were the overpronator's kiss of death. Even orthotics could not correct overpronation when used in conjunction with soft midsoles. As the orthotic sank into the shoebed, correction was lost. Because no hard-sole running shoes were being sold, we even recommended conventional walking shoes with rigid crepe soles, which provided a firm platform and eliminated excess roll-over to the sides. As shoe manufacturers began receiving recommendations from various sportsmedicine podiatrists, there began a small trend back to shoes with greater foot control. While we have seen the change, the percentage of soft- to firm-soled shoes is still wrong. About 80 percent of all runners need control with hard-soled shoes and 20 percent need cushioning due to high-arched feet; however, we have 80 percent of the shoes providing lots of cushioning — good for high-arched feet — and only 20 percent of the shoes providing stability for the pronators.

I know you would like to see us recommend a particular shoe. Unfortunately, shoe brands and styles change with the wind. A shoe we are currently recommending for the overpronator is slowly being pulled off the market. Fortunately others are coming up to take its place.

If you have high-arched feet, your choice of shoe is not difficult. You can probably wear any shoe that is comfortable and gives adequate cushioning to prevent shock absorption problems — your No. 1 enemy. The air-soled shoes are recommended. For overpronators, we recommend hard-soled shoes, which helps overpronation. Many running shoe ads promote control through the heel counter; we feel that the heel counter has little to do with control.

As explained earlier, heelstrike is at the back, outside corner.

Body weight is distributed from there forward along the outside to approximately midarch, where it traverses the ball of the foot and finally out the big toe. If you have a soft midsole and you are an overpronator, after forefoot contact is made, you will continue to pronate; the medial side of the shoe continues to compress. This will accentuate problems stemming from overpronation. Softer midsoles also have a shorter shoe life, approximately five hundred miles — or less. They begin to compress in the area of greatest stress, usually the inside part of the shoe. This once again contributes to overpronation. When a runner does not overpronate but lands on the outside of the foot and remains on the outside of the foot, his shoe will compress here. As a result, lateral knee or leg pain can often develop.

Fortunately, strengthening the heel between the midsole and the heel counter on the inside will help eliminate overpronation in some shoes. Some of the shoes made this way are providing both excellent cushioning ability and control.

INNERSOLES

There are two basic methods of innersole construction. One is cement lasting, whereby the upper- and midsole are cemented to an intermediate, fiberboard sheet. The other method is slip lasting, whereby the upper is sewn into the midsole and no fiberboard is used. The slip-lasted shoe is much more flexible than the fiberboard shoe. An orthotic used with a slip-lasted shoe might allow excessive pronation, especially if the shoe is made with a soft midsole.

In the cement-lasted shoe, the insole board — a flat piece of cellulose fiber — is treated with chemicals to help combat bacteria and fungus.

On top of the insole board is glued a sock liner made of foam rubber, crushed velour, terry cloth, and sometimes Spenco. The liner helps absorb sweat, impact, and prevent blisters. Based on our case studies, we find that the terry cloth innersole promotes blisters and gives little protection from impact. The Spenco innersole, on the other hand, is superior in both respects. Spenco, a closed-cell material that resists flattening over a long period, also accommodates lateral movement, which helps prevent blisters. If you have a sock liner in your shoe, we suggest that it be removed and replaced with a Spenco innersole.

Arch Supports

Most sports shoes will have, underneath the sock liner, a wedge-shaped piece of foam called an arch cookie. This is put here to give arch support, but does nothing more than make for a slightly snug fit. In many of the newer running shoes, there are variations on the theme of a built-in orthotic or arch support. Some of these work admirably, whereas others are merely formed foam to fit the footbed and quickly compress so as to be worthless. If you feel that you need some type of arch support and purchase a shoe with a built-in support system, do not immediately wear the shoe on a long run. Wear the shoe for a couple hours around the house the first day, increasing by an hour per day for ten days. Then you may begin running a couple miles, increasing by a mile every other day until you have become accustomed to the support. The process compares to getting used to wearing contact lenses; that is, you do not wear them all day the first few days.

Whenever prescription orthotics are purchased for your running shoes, be sure to remove any support system or formed padding that comes with the shoes. The orthotic needs a flat bed. An arch cookie left in the shoe may be placed too far forward; in this position it will lift up the front part of the orthotic, and make wearing them quite uncomfortable. To avoid problems, bring your running shoes when you visit the podiatrist to get your orthotics so that he can make the necessary alterations in your shoes.

Heel Counter

This plastic or fiberboard stiffener built into the heel of the shoe supposedly helps prevent the foot from rolling too far to the inside during the gait cycle, thus eliminating overpronation. When you consider the forces involved with footstrike, however, the heel counter can't do much more than provide support for the shoe upper. Just above the heel counter you will usually find a tab of padded vinyl, which is utilized to protect the Achilles tendon and to give a fingerhold when you slip on your shoes. Occasionally this tab will irritate a runner's Achilles tendon. To reduce that possibility we suggest that socks be worn high enough to act as a buffer between the Achilles tendon and the tab.

SHOE UPPER

Shoe uppers are made from many different materials — leather, nylon, Gore-Tex, canvas. Most shoe uppers are made from nylon, with leather foxing reinforcing the toebox and heel counter area. Nylon is light and pliable, desirable characteristics in a shoe upper.

When selecting running shoes, make sure that the leather surrounding that toebox rides far enough over the top of your toes. The point where the leather and nylon meet should not be where your toenails touch. Toenails can easily rub on this edge, increasing shoe wear here, or worse, irritate or tear away a toenail. Breathability varies with different nylon fabrics, but distinguishing which shoe material breathes better than another can only be determined with first-hand experience. Upper material that breathes poorly can cause foot discomfort and make feet more susceptible to blistering from increased temperatures. Here are some more pointers concerning shoes and shoe care:

- There are many variations of lacing. Some women find that lacing that extends around the heel counter gives extra support for narrow heels.

- A shoe with a cutout in the tongue, which allows laces to go through, will prevent the tongue from sliding around.

- Never wash your shoes in a washing machine or put them into a dryer to dry. If your shoes are dirty, wash them with a damp washcloth and let them air dry.

- Never put your shoes by a furnace or heating duct and do not leave them in the sun; the outer sole may come unglued and separate from the midsole.

- Before a run, always inspect your shoes for fraying, holes, excessive wear, or separation.

- *Runner's World* magazine has published numerous shoe studies by Peter Cavanagh, professor of biomechanics at Pennsylvania State University. They are interesting and valuable reading.

15

Orthotics

Orthotics are one of the mainstays in preventing injuries to the active person. Orthotics do not treat the symptoms of injury, they treat the cause. Therefore, their use is extremely beneficial when dealing with injuries caused by foot imbalances.

No piece of equipment available to the active person is more misunderstood than the orthotic. We want to make it clear here that not everyone needs orthotics. They are not a panacea and should not be thought of as such. Orthotics work well for specific problems only if the proper examination is made and the orthotic device is properly constructed. The following question- and-answer format is used to answer the many queries we receive about orthotics.

What is an orthotic?

An orthotic is a prescription device constructed to accommodate an individual's feet, which corrects abnormal foot biomechanics. They are made of various materials, sometimes molded plastic, leather or other similar material. A pair can be worn comfortably in either running or street shoes.

Aren't orthotics just exotic, expensive arch supports?

No. This is a popular fallacy about orthotics. Arch supports are soft, pliable inserts you can purchase at drugstores. These cushion the feet, but do not control abnormal forces in your gait. Arch supports are mass-produced so that the few sizes made will fit all feet. Orthotics, on the other hand, are custom-made by your podiatrist.

How are orthotics made?

A cast of each foot is made using plaster. Information is also gleaned from X-rays and a biomechanical range-of-motion examination before the orthotic is constructed. Sometimes the shape of a pair of orthotics varies between each foot as a result of biomechanical differences.

How much difference is there between cushioning and controlling abnormal foot function?

Plenty. A foot that functions abnormally will be unable to handle the stresses that are generated at each step, particularly when subjected to a sports activity. An orthotic may be necessary for proper support. A soft, cushioning arch support is not rigid enough for the task. Even if you made your own orthotic out of a rigid material, it probably would not be comfortable enough to wear. That's why we take a mold of the foot, so that the orthotic will conform and feel comfortable. A slight variation in the required shape will result in abnormal footstrike, which is why rigid orthotics are not sold without a prescription.

But isn't a rigid orthotic going to be uncomfortable in the shoe?

Definitely not. But it must be made properly. After getting used to wearing rigid orthotics, you sometimes forget they're in your shoe. Very few athletes have problems with comfort. In fact, many orthotic wearers say that going without them causes a strange sensation in the feet, as though their feet were collapsing, which indeed they are.

Does the orthotic change the shape of the foot?

No. Orthotics accommodate the foot and allow it to function normally by placing it in its neutral position. The actual anatomical structure of the foot will not be changed. In other words, if you have a flat foot, it will not go away by wearing orthotics. The use of orthotics can be compared to wearing glasses. Just as wearing glasses will not anatomically correct eyesight, wearing orthotics will not anatomically correct footstrike.

Isn't a flat foot just a collapsed arch?

It isn't that simple. A collapsed arch is only part of the problem. A flat foot is an overpronated foot. The overpronated foot better describes the flat foot dilemma. The heel of the overpronated foot spends the majority of its time everted during the gait cycle, as shown in Fig. 3-1. The arch collapses because the muscles that normally hold it up are strained and weakened.

How do you get pronated feet?

This is usually determined by genetics. A serious injury could also result in overpronation. If there is a tendency in your family to have overpronated feet, you will have similar problems.

So orthotics put the feet in their neutral position?

That's right. Fig. 3-1 shows a person standing who has overpronated feet. We then show this same individual standing in orthotics. This position will allow the foot to function normally about its neutral position.

How can I tell if I have a flat foot?

Sometimes that can be quite difficult. Many problems are subtle and require podiatric evaluation. A good indicator of abnormal foot function, however, is shoe wear. We tend not to put too much importance in shoe wear on the bottom of the shoe. Most people tend to wear out their shoes in the same pattern – on the outside heel and inside ball of the foot. More important is the relationship of the heel to the ground. Fig. 3-3 demonstrates this relationship. A new shoe heel will be perpendicular to the surface. Over time, if the foot functions normally about its neutral position, the heel of the shoe will remain stationary. However, with abnormal footstrike, the heel area of the shoe "forms" to accommodate the abnormal position of the foot. At least it looks that way, as you will see in Fig. 3-4, which shows the shoes of a runner with severe flat feet. These shoes are only three months old. Note the extreme wear pattern caused by the heel being forced into maximum pronation.

Does every active person need orthotics?

No. A lot of people have feet that function properly, or that might be slightly abnormal but still cause no trouble. Every injury is not caused by bad feet.

Will orthotics solve all my activity-related injury problems?

As we already stated, orthotics are not a panacea. For example, a severely painful injury that causes your knee to unlock, give out or swell might not be the typical runner's knee caused by foot imbalances. Severe problems require orthopedic consultation; there could be something seriously wrong with the knee joint. Common sense prevails.

If I'm an active person who needs orthotics, what should I expect from my doctor?

X-ray evaluation, gait analysis, casting, recommendations for shoe gear, and follow-up care are the basics. A medical history will be taken. If you have a foot dysfunction, the doctor should explain the problem and how orthotics will correct it. The podiatrist should watch you walk or run in order to see how your foot, leg, knee and pelvis function. X-rays are taken to determine the bone structure of your feet. A range-of-motion exam is performed to measure the amount of motion available in the various joints of the foot and leg. After this, a cast is taken of each foot. The doctor should do the casting, not a member of his office staff. The casting is the most important step in making orthotics.

Do most podiatrists know what they are doing?

Those involved with sportsmedicine do. To be sure, ask other runners who know podiatrists to recommend.

What is the cost of orthotics?

The fee ranges from $150 to more than $400. Sometimes, however, price quotes can be misleading. There are several steps in preparing a patient for orthotics — casting, X-rays, biomechanical exam, gait analysis. When you get a price quote, find out exactly what the fee includes and what it does not include. Check your health insurance to see if orthotics are covered. Most insurance companies will pay for orthotics.

What if my feet don't hurt. Do I still need orthotics?

Possibly. Undue stress from abnormal footstrike affects not only the foot, but leg and body. These stresses can cause runner's knee, shinsplints, heel pain, hip/back pain and more. Yet the feet may not hurt.

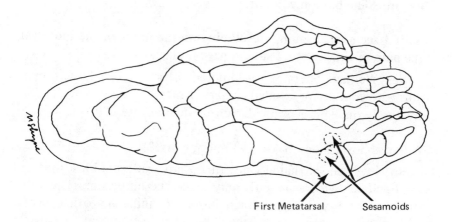

First Metatarsal   Sesamoids

Fig. 15-1 Bones of Foot with Bunion

Some doctors opposed to orthotics say that if your feet don't hurt, you needn't treat them. However, the debilitating effect of age can be accelerated if a body imbalance is ignored. Treatment is sometimes instituted even if it doesn't hurt at the time.

What are bunions and will orthotics help correct them?

Bunions are caused primarily by pronated or flat feet. A large tendon that attaches to the base of the big toe pulls the big toe, which in turn pushes the first metatarsal head out. A large bump, which is typical of a bunion, forms. Fig. 15-1 shows a full-blown deformity.

An incipient to moderate-size bunion is usually painless. The deformity occurs over a span of many years. Over time, the first metatarsal joint will adapt to the new position of the big toe. This can eventually lead to erosion of the cartilage, and then pain and arthritis.

How does the orthotic help?

Once the bunion is set, there is little that can be done other than surgery. The bones are set in their new position and they must be realigned. The orthotic will not change what's already there. However, a developing bunion can be arrested by an ortho-tic, which controls the abnormal forces that allowed the bunion to form. The bunion will not, however, go away.

So if I see a small bump developing on the inside of the foot near the base of the big toe, I should have it checked?

Yes. We have operated on hundreds of active people with bun-ions who could have avoided surgery if they had only seen a podia-trist early on. This is particularly true in children.

Will my sports shoes make the bunion worse?

No. Even shoes that do not fit do not cause bunions; that's a myth. Shoes with a poor fit only make the bunion more painful from pressure on the prominent bump. Running and other sports with a lot of movement hasten bunion development, however.

What about my shoes accommodating orthotics?

Most shoes will accommodate orthotics without any problem. However, a heavily padded shoe sole will allow the orthotic to compress the heel, which leads to instability.

Do I wear orthotics only when I'm involved in my sport?

No. They should be worn the majority of the day in your work shoes. You can't, however, wear orthotics in high-heel or open-toed shoes.

Do I wear the orthotics the rest of my life?

Yes, if you want to maintain proper footstrike. They are dur-able and rarely break.

Will my shoes wear longer?

Yes, because abnormal footstrike is neutralized and so is ab-normal wear.

Are there different kinds of orthotics?

Yes. We generally classify them according to rigidity: There are rigid, semi-rigid and soft orthotics. The rigidity of orthotic pre-scribed depends on such factors as your age, sport activity, and footstrike abnormality. Many doctors make their own orthotics rather than order them from a specialty lab. We have found that specialty labs make the best orthotics. They also offer greater variety.

What long-term problems have you seen with orthotics?

If the orthotic is made properly and is the right one for the individual, none. However, a poorly made orthotic will cause more problems. One patient who saw us had a box full of orthotics, from leather to steel. All were poorly constructed, and the patient continued having problems until we fitted her with the proper quality orthotic.

We do not recommend purchasing orthotics through the mail or in any retail store. Some people have been injured by using them.

16

Medications

It is not our intention here to imply that medications should be used for every problem. We avoid the use of drugs. It is wise to avoid using a drug, which will course through the entire body, to treat minor injuries that can be corrected by localized, non-invasive methods. But there are circumstances where medications are indicated.

Why are drugs necessary at all, you might ask? Because some drugs are effective at controlling inflammation. By controlling inflammation after an injury, the healing process is enhanced.

There are thousands of drugs on the market whose function is to reduce inflammation. We will discuss several of the more common ones and what to expect when these drugs are used. We emphasize that you should not think that "a pill for every problem" is an appropriate attitude. Drugs are just one alternative to bring about quick healing and a return to activity. We first try ice, heat or other modalities. Some doctors will prescribe a drug to every patient no matter what the severity of the injury. We feel this is wrong.

ASPIRIN

Aspirin is the most widely used over-the-counter drug in the world. It is quite effective in aiding the repair of injury by reducing the symptoms of inflammation. It was first used by the Ancient

Romans, who took it from the lining of tree bark. It was originally used to reduce fever, and still is today. Aspirin will reduce any elevated body temperature, but will not change a normal body temperature.

Aspirin has more recently been recognized for its properties as a mild analgesic. Aspirin's analgesic effect is not strong enough to mask pain to the point that it is no longer felt. If you have a bad case of shinsplints and take aspirin before a run, it will not enable you to run pain-free.

The most important property of aspirin for the athlete is its ability to reduce inflammation. The drug can be taken in fairly high doses with minimal side effects, which makes aspirin a quite safe medication. Some people, however, are allergic to aspirin. If we prescribe aspirin, we recommend taking two tablets every four to six hours. This amount is usually prescribed for a fairly severe injury or strain during the acute phase of healing. That usually amounts to the first few days or week after injury. We do not recommend taking aspirin for extended periods.

Some people have problems with aspirin causing an upset stomach. To rectify this problem, you can take aspirin that contains Maalox, which settles the stomach.

Aspirin may also be effective during the secondary stage of healing, the time when training resumes at a reduced level. We recommend taking two aspirin about a half-hour before the activity is commenced. The reason for taking aspirin before you run is that when you start working out it will already be in your system. When you are running, the majority of your blood is in the lower extremity. So the injured area is "washed" with the anti-inflammatory medication. Use aspirin sparingly. We discourage aspirin use on a regular basis when there is no injury present.

NON-STEROIDAL ANTI-INFLAMMATORIES

Non-steroidal anti-inflammatories do not contain cortisone or cortisone-like derivatives. Non-steroidal, anti-inflammatory medications include such drugs as Indocin, Butazolidin, Naprosyn, Motrin, Tolectin and other similar compounds. These drugs are specifically manufactured to reduce inflammation. They are not analgesics nor do they have any other related properties, as does aspirin. Also, they are of varying strengths. In our experience, Butazolidin tends to be the strongest, while Tolectin seems to be the weakest. We can prescribe an individual an anti-inflammatory geared to the severity of the injury. If you have a severe ankle sprain, for instance, then we might prescribe Butazolidin for a couple of days. On the other hand, for mild shinsplints, Motrin might be helpful. Most of these drugs, because they are stronger than aspirin, have a greater potential for side effects. However, we have found that by using these medications for a short time, say three to six days, the side effects are minimal. Most common of the side effects is a mildly upset stomach, which can be overcome by taking the drugs with milk or food. These drugs, because they are not cortisone derivatives and because they are non-narcotic, do not have any deleterious side effects like drowsiness.

CORTISONE

Cortisone has such a reputation that it is misunderstood by most athletes. What is cortisone and what does it do? Cortisone is the strongest known anti-inflammatory medication. It is grouped under the heading of compounds known as steroids. Steroids are chemicals produced by the body in the adrenal glands. They have a myriad of functions, from producing sexual characteristics to controlling protein, carbohydrate and fat metabolism. Moreover, certain steroids have the unique property of being strongly anti-inflammatory. According to Goodman and Gilman in their pharmacology text, cortisone "at the microscopic level, inhibits not only the early phenomena of the inflammatory process but also the latter manifestations."

Cortisone can be taken orally or through injection. The side effects of this drug are many, which is why it has such a bad reputation. These side effects include cataracts, loss of bone density, acne, moon face, suppression of the adrenal gland function and other bizarre side effects. But these side effects only occur when high doses are taken for a prolonged time.

An injection of a few drops of cortisone into an injured area will not cause the described side effects. When taken for a long time, however, the adrenal glands sense an increase in cortisone in the body and respond by reducing their output of steroids. This is, in a sense, an addiction; the body needs the cortisone that is being supplied to it every day. Therefore, when cortisone use is discontinued, it must be done gradually so that the adrenal glands can gradually increase production of the natural steroids.

Not every injury requires cortisone. Indeed, we have had patients come to us who were injected more than ten times in the same area and had no alleviation of symptoms. That number of shots is obviously gross drug abuse.

Cortisone, however, has its place in medical use, but it must be treated with respect. A single injection of cortisone into an injured area is not abusing the drug.

There are many other "drugs" used commonly by doctors of sportsmedicine. For instance, many people feel that vitamin supplements play an active role in the treatment and prevention of injury. This may be true, but it is up to the individual to decide.

17

Surgery

Surgeons must be very careful
When they take the knife!
Underneath their fine incisions
Stirs the culprit — life!
  — Emily Dickinson

Any book on foot care would be incomplete without a discussion of surgical procedures on the foot and ankle. What we have attempted to present in this book is how to recognize, treat, and prevent injuries in the active person. We also have attempted to clarify when and when not to seek professional help and try self-treatment methods, and to discuss injuries specific to individual activities. It has been our intention to thoroughly examine the foot, its motions, and its surrounding structure so that the individual can understand the workings of his or her own foot. We also have shown how the foot, ankle and leg in proper motion can relate to the overall health of the body and maintenance of injury-free activity.

In order to complete the picture of total foot care, it is necessary to discuss surgery as an alternative treatment. It must be remembered, and it will be emphasized over and over again in this chapter, that surgery should be considered a final alternative. It should never be considered the initial treatment, or even a secondary or tertiary treatment, but rather only a last resort. Conversely, surgery *is* an alternative when all conservative treatments have failed.

Although foot surgery is not classified as "life threatening," one imagines potential foot surgery as fraught with risks, including a prolonged recovery period and the possibility of continual foot pain after surgery interfering with normal activity. Unfortunately, this fallacious image is locked in the minds of the general public — an image supported by what we have come to call "horror stories" of surgery performed on the feet of friends and relatives. It is not uncommon for a potential surgical patient to come to us prior to surgery and say, "Mrs. Jones had this surgery and has never been the same." It is certainly true that many people in the past have suffered needlessly from improper foot surgery. New techniques, however, have been developed in the last several years that have made foot surgery safe, simple, inexpensive and, more important, effective without long-term complications.

One major problem with foot surgery as opposed to other types of surgery is that the foot-surgery patient must be able to walk at the surgical site. This is much different than having surgery, say, on the hand or face — structures that don't have the weight-bearing function of feet. The foot, on the other hand, comes in contact with Mother Earth first, and the surgery must take into consideration the time needed for the area to heal properly and, at the same time, allow the patient to ambulate normally — a fine balance to maintain. Foot surgery, therefore, unlike other surgical procedures, must be performed with great precision and care. The proper surgical procedure must be selected and surgery should be performed only when necessary. In our surgical practice, we perform a large number of "re-do" surgeries (surgeries other doctors did). In many cases, these previous surgeries were either unnecessary or poorly executed. Foot surgery is a delicate art and must be approached as such.

The purpose of this chapter is to discuss the new information available on foot surgery and to prepare a foot-surgery patient for what will occur before, during and after the operation. It is imperative for the patient to be aware of what will take place. We have found that an informed, prepared patient copes with surgery and the post-surgical period much better than an uninformed one.

NECESSITY FOR SURGERY

Perhaps the most important question to ask about foot surgery is, "Is the surgery really necessary?" Many of our patients believe that surgery is the only option they have to correct their particular problem. In most cases, other, more conservative, non-invasive treatments can be first attempted to rectify a given problem. It is a rare instance that surgery is the only treatment available. We almost always tell our patients, "We can always do surgery if necessary, but let's try something more conservative first." Most patients welcome the opportunity to have various treatments explained to them, and to be given a choice in the matter. If the more conservative treatments fail, however, or if the individual desires surgery, then he or she must be made aware of what will transpire.

ABOUT THE SURGERY

Once you have decided to undergo surgery, you should consider several factors. First, and most important, you should understand what is being done and why. It seems obvious to ask your doctor, but many patients go into surgery completely oblivious to what's going on. The concepts of surgery are not difficult to grasp. Ask your doctor to explain with models, drawings or X-rays exactly what will be done and why. It should make sense to you why something will be performed in a given manner. If it doesn't make sense or your doctor is reluctant to explain, we suggest finding another surgeon or get a second opinion. There must be a reason your doctor won't explain, whether because of poor past performances or personality problems.

At this point, a word about communication is in order. Remember that you are placing your body in the hands of what is, in most cases, a total stranger. You must have an open line of communication with your doctor and you must feel comfortable with his or her abilities. If your doctor talks down to you, doesn't talk at all, or seems aloof, and you're uncomfortable with him, then we would suggest finding another doctor. We have found that one of the biggest causes of an unhappy patient is a breakdown in communication with the doctor. In some instances, this line of communication has never been established, or the doctor has failed to communicate adequately. If you are uncomfortable with your doctor prior to surgery, you will still be uncomfortable after surgery, which could lead to problems. Again, seek someone you feel comfortable with.

QUALIFICATIONS

Make sure your surgeon is well-trained to do the surgery. Don't assume your doctor knows how to perform the procedure just because he is a doctor. Many doctors do a minimal amount of surgery, and you may be taking a chance with someone who is not qualified to perform a particular operation. The question then arises, "How does one determine how well-qualified the surgeon is?"

We strongly recommend consulting a podiatric surgeon, who is an expert on the foot and foot surgery, since this is all he or she does. Not every podiatrist is a surgeon, however. Find one who has an active, well-established, hospital-based surgical practice. Surgeons who perform poorly tend not to survive. Contact your hospital or local medical society to find out who is well-trained in your area. You can also consult the American Board of Podiatric Surgery, which certifies the better-qualified surgeons. To be qualified, a podiatrist must have been in active practice for several years, performed a certain number of representative hospital surgeries and passed lengthy written and oral exams.

Another important aspect about your surgeon is his or her track record. How well has he performed in the past? One way to determine this is to ask your surgeon to give you names of patients he has operated on. You can then contact several patients who have undergone similar operations to ask, first of all, how the surgery went, and secondly, specific questions about what will take place. Again, most doctors should be willing to provide you with names of former patients. If he or she is reluctant, we would again suggest switching surgeons. Remember, in the final analysis, it's your body being operated on, and you have the right to know what qualifications your surgeon has and what to expect from the surgery. As a patient, you should demand this information.

ANESTHESIA

The word anesthesia comes from the Greek word meaning to have loss of feeling or sensation. The "best" anesthesia makes the patient comfortable and, at the same time, makes it easy for the surgeon to perform a given operation. Several forms of anesthesia are available, but we will just discuss local and general anesthesia.

Local anesthesia is probably the safest anesthesia available. An injection given by your dentist is an example of a "local." The anesthetic is injected directly into the surgical area, which causes a temporary cessation of nerve impulses to that area. There are several advantages to a local. Since the patient is awake and only the surgical area is numb, there is little risk of complications. In addition, the patient isn't groggy after the operation, so the surgery can be performed either in the office or as an outpatient in the hospital.

Locals, however, also have several disadvantages. Since the patient is awake, he may be more apprehensive, which increases the possibility of his feeling sick or faint. Also, the injection may be uncomfortable and time-consuming. If the surgical site is large, getting anesthesia to the entire area may be difficult, and there may be pain during the procedure. If the patient and doctor feel that the disadvantages outweigh the advantages of a local anesthesia, then a general anesthesia is advised.

With general anesthesia, the patient is completely asleep. General anesthesia is comfortable for the patient and convenient for the surgeon. The patient is usually given a pre-operative sedative, and once in the operating room, an intravenous line is established. When everything is set, sodium pentathol is injected into the patient via the intravenous line. Sodium pentathol acts quickly – in a matter of seconds. The patient feels only a relaxing and comfortable sleep. Once the sodium pentathol takes effect, gaseous anesthesia is administered and the operation begins. After surgery, the patient wakes up slowly, taking anywhere from several minutes to an hour.

Complications from general anesthesia are rare, and when they do occur, extenuating circumstances, such as the patient's general poor health, are usually to blame. With proper pre-operative screening for elective surgery, general anesthesia is almost totally risk-free.

Regardless of the type of anesthesia used, the important point to keep in mind is patient comfort. As previously stated, the patient and the surgeon must mutually decide on the anesthesia to be administered.

HOSPITAL VS. OFFICE SURGERY

This is a controversial issue, one that has elicited a myriad of opinions. Some surgeons perform all of their surgery, from the simplest to the most complicated, in the office. Others do all their procedures in the hospital, no matter how simple the operation. We believe that some procedures can be performed in the office, and other, more complicated, surgeries should be reserved for the hospital. The hospital provides constant, professional care, and the operating rooms are far better equipped and more sterile than those in the office. Moreover, various forms of anesthesia are available in the hospital, while in the office, only a local injection can be given. We operate on toes and simple bunions in the office, but we feel that many other procedures require the safety and services of a hospital. In most cases, the patient need only register as an outpatient to receive podiatric surgery, and since there is no need to stay overnight, it is much less expensive.

In the surgical community, particularly among podiatrists, minimal incision surgery (MIS) is gaining popularity. In this type of surgery, a local anesthetic is used and a tiny stab incision is made in the skin. A high-speed, cutting burr is then inserted into the foot, and surgery is performed until the desired correction is obtained. There is nothing wrong with MIS when it's properly used for the appropriate procedure. Although it seems to be getting a lot of publicity lately, we have been performing MIS in the office for years.

POST-OPERATIVE COURSE

By far, the most common post-operative question patients ask is, "When will I be able to walk normally again?" In all honesty, we tell them that it is difficult to determine exactly when. We state an average time, however, since from our experience, each individual responds differently to a given surgical procedure. We take into consideration the extent of the surgery, what part of the foot was operated on, the patient's age, amount of activity immediately after surgery, and recuperative abilities. Many factors, therefore, go into determining exactly when someone will be able to resume normal activity.

We should make it clear, however, that in the majority of cases, the patient is able to walk the same evening after surgery is performed. Casts are rarely required, as are any external fixations like pins. The patient ambulates by means of a wooden post-operative shoe. We strongly discourage the use of crutches, walkers or wheelchairs, for two reasons. First, with the advent of new surgical techniques, these devices are unnecessary, and second, it's important that the patient not become dependent on crutches or a walker. By permitting them to move, the legs and feet stay strong and the healing process is accelerated. Therefore, we find that ambulation immediately after surgery is beneficial, with minimal discomfort.

On the average, most patients who undergo moderate surgery like a bunionectomy are able to return to work within a week afterward. In most cases, the patient is back into normal shoe gear and ambulating painlessly in four to six weeks after the procedure.

In summary, post-operative healing involves many considerations. By controlling these various factors, however, we have found that the majority of foot-surgery patients respond quickly, adequately, with minimal discomfort and are able to return to normal activity.

FOOT PROCEDURES

Bunions

Bunions are probably the most common foot ailment requiring surgery. A bunion is formed by a complex imbalance within the foot, and is usually caused by overpronation, which we discussed in Chapter 3. Fig. 17-1a shows an X-ray of a typical bunion. Note that the joint is displaced and the big toe is drifting toward the lesser toes. Every bunion deformity is different. In many cases, the bunion on the right foot of an individual will be different from the one on the left. There are hundreds of procedures that can be performed on bunions, and it's up to your doctor to determine which procedure is appropriate for your problem. Fig. 17-1b shows a post-operative X-ray of the bunion pictured in Fig. 17-1a. Note that the toes are straight and the foot looks normal.

New bunion procedures developed recently have had excellent long-term results. The use of implant surgery to replace arthritic or destroyed joints is also relatively new and has become a highly successful, pain-free operation. The implant is made of a pliable, plastic material that doesn't break and presents no allergic problems. We have used these implants many times with no long-term complications. In fact, the implants work so well that many patients are amazed by how quickly they recover and how completely their previous pain is assuaged.

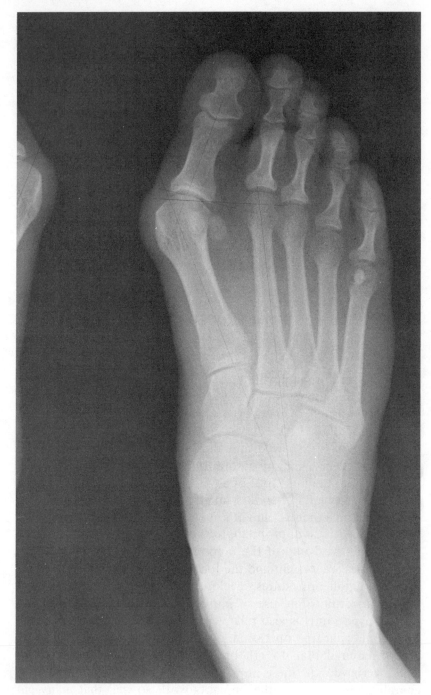

Fig. 17-1a *An X-ray of a typical bunion.*

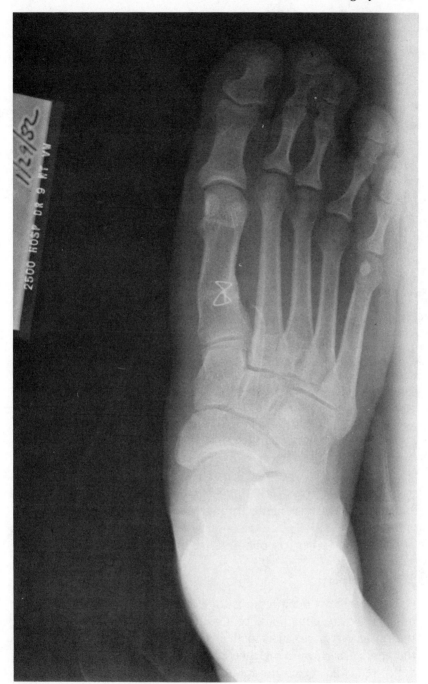

Fig. 17-1b *The same foot, one year after corrective surgery.*

Hammertoes

A hammertoe is a toe that is cocked up, as shown in Fig. 17-2. The causes of hammertoes include improper shoe gear, previous injury, high-arched feet, bunions, Morton's toe (where the second toe is the longest), and others that were previously discussed. No matter what the cause, hammertoes can be quite a problem since most develop a painful corn on the top of the toe. If all efforts at self-treatment fail, surgical correction is necessary; it can be performed in the office under a local anesthetic. Surgery consists of removing the portion of bone at the high point of the deformity. Fig. 17-3 shows a diagrammatic representation of a toe before and after surgery. The toe is slightly less functional after surgery, but it's not noticeable to the patient. After the operation, the toe is straight and the pain is gone.

Recuperation takes anywhere from several days to several weeks. Normal, loose-fitting shoes can be worn after several days, and most people are back to their normal activities within two to three weeks.

Heel Spurs

As discussed previously, heel spurs are a common affliction among active people. As you will recall, however, the name "heel spur" is a misnomer. The heel spur is a secondary problem. The root of the ailment is a pull of the plantar fascia from the heel bone. Because 99 percent of all heel spurs clear up with conservative treatment, surgery is rarely prescribed. When attempted, surgery removes the spur and cuts the plantar fascia. In theory, the plantar fascia grows back longer when it reattaches to the heel bone. The incison is made through the side of the foot, and a cast may be applied. Healing takes several weeks, and the success rate is good. Remember, try conservative therapy before surgery.

Toenail Surgery

There are two main reasons for performing nail surgery: to clear up an ingrown toenail, and to eliminate fungus nails. In both cases, the surgery is performed in the office under a local anesthetic. In the case of a chronic ingrown nail, only the offending side or border is removed. Once the nail is removed, the cells that grow that particular portion of the nail are destroyed, either with acid, a burr, a surgical scalpel, or another method. We have found surgery to be the best. The toe heals within a couple of days.

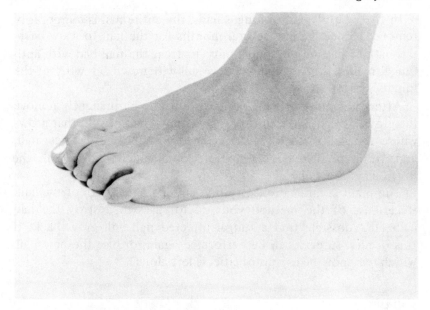

Fig. 17-2 *Hammertoes result from a variety of causes.*

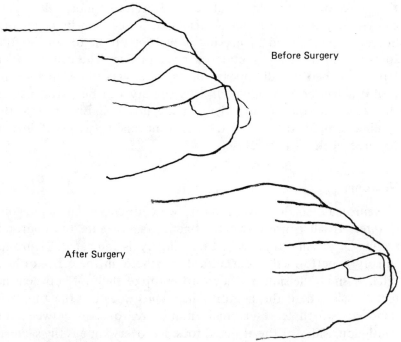

Before Surgery

After Surgery

Fig. 17-3 Hammertoes

In the case of painful fungus nails, the entire nail is temporarily removed. Since it takes several months for the nail to grow back, the patient has ample opportunity to treat the nail bed with anti-fungal medication so that the new nail will grow back without the fungus.

After the nail is off, the other option is to permanently remove the growth cells. The result is a small, tough bed of skin that grows where the nail once was. This skin looks almost like a new nail, and from a cosmetic standpoint, looks much better than the previously infected nail.

The main complication with this surgery is regrowth of the nail. Regardless of the method your doctor uses to destroy the nail cells, it's possible that a fungal infected nail will grow back. If this occurs, surgery can be performed again, or else the new nail, which may now be asymptomatic, is left alone.

Calluses

If a patient is tired of a painful callus on the bottom of the foot, or of trimming down the callus every month, surgery can be performed to correct the problem permanently. With callus surgery, the source of the problem is attacked. Recall that most calluses are caused by a metatarsal that is displaced lower than its neighbors. Surgery is performed by making an incision on the top of the foot to raise the displaced metatarsal back in line. The callus is then left untouched and disappears on its own, since the source of the problem has been eliminated. This surgery can be performed in the office or on an outpatient in the hospital. Either way, the healing is rapid; the person returns to normal activity within two to three weeks after surgery.

Neuromas

Neuromas, small nerve tumors, were discussed in a previous chapter. If all conservative treatments fail to cure the neuroma (which is usually the case), then surgery is indicated. Neuroma surgery is performed under a local anesthetic in the office or hospital. A small incision is made on the top of the foot between the metatarsals where the neuroma lies. Once located, the tumor is removed, which leaves a small, numb area of skin between the contiguous sides of the affected toes. Recovery time is the same as with other forefoot operations — two to four weeks.

OTHER SURGICAL PROCEDURES

We have discussed the more common surgeries performed on the foot, but there are hundreds of other routine surgeries that will not be discussed in detail here. If you have any problems that you think might require surgery, consult your podiatrist to learn exactly what should be done. Remember, when it comes to surgery of the foot, your podiatrist is the expert.

SURGICAL FEES

With the rising costs of medical care today, many patients are concerned about the cost of surgery. The cost of the operation, however, should not be the deciding factor on who should do the surgery. Again, pick a qualified surgeon. Most doctors in a given area will charge about the same fee for a particular procedure. Before the surgery, get an estimate of fees to determine exactly how much the surgery will cost. Submit it to your insurance company prior to the surgery, and you can determine how much it will pay. Any doctor will give you such an estimate. You can also check with other doctors to find out if you are being charged too much, but we advise you not to make the fee the deciding factor. Financial considerations are certainly important, but your most important consideration is getting a qualified surgeon.

In summary, foot surgery has over the last decade become a refined science. The old stories of patients crippled by foot surgery are no longer true if the surgery is performed properly. Remember, surgery should be an alternative, not the only option, but if it is decided upon, realize that it is safe, relatively pain-free, and will allow you to function without any discomfort. We have included at the end of this chapter several points to ask your doctor prior to contemplating foot surgery. It's your body being operated upon, and you have every right to know what will transpire before, during and after a foot operation.

POINTS TO ASK OF YOUR DOCTOR PRIOR TO SURGERY

1) Have the doctor thoroughly explain what the problem is. Don't just assume he or she knows what's going on. Have a basic idea of what caused the problem and why. If need be, look at your

X-rays to help understand the problem. Ask your doctor what you can read to expand your knowledge of the potential surgery.

2) Understand exactly what the surgical procedure consists of. How big is the incision and where will it be placed? What structures (tendon, bone, etc.) will be involved? X-rays, models and drawings make this task easy. Surgical procedures are simple for the most part, and one should be able to grasp easily what will take place.

3) What anesthesia will be used? Let the doctor know your preferences, and be sure you understand the different anesthesias available. Respect the doctor's opinion based on his or her experience. Remember that the best anesthesia makes the patient comfortable and allows the surgeon ease in performing the operation.

4) Have the recovery period laid out for you, or at least have a general idea of what will happen after the surgery. When can you walk? When do the stitches come out? Can you drive? How much pain will you have? In most instances, the surgeon will be unable to give you exact answers to these questions since every individual is unique. But you should be able to get a rough idea of what to expect during the recovery period.

5) Understand the potential complications. Although they are rare, you don't want to be totally shocked if something should go wrong.

6) If you're not 100 percent sure about the diagnosis or the doctor's ability, get another opinion. Surgery is elective, and you usually have the time to get a second or third evaluation. Seek a board-certified or board-eligible podiatric surgeon — he or she is the best trained to perform foot surgery.

7) Ask about fees for reference purposes only; don't make this a major consideration in deciding who will do the surgery. Remember that shopping around for the least expensive surgeon can lead to disaster.

8) Ask about the long-term effects of the surgery. What will happen in one year? Five years? Twenty years? Will the problem return? Again, prepare yourself for what's to come.

About the Authors

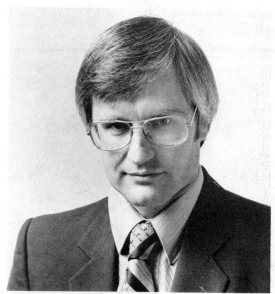

Dennis R. Zamzow, D.P.M.

Dennis R. Zamzow is a native of Ripon, Wisconsin. He currently resides in Cupertino, California, and is in private practice in Mountain View, California. He is a staff member of El Camino Hospital in Mountain View and Valley West Hospital in Los Gatos, California. He served in the Navy from 1962 to 1970 as an inertial navigation, computer and electronics technician aboard the nuclear-powered Polaris missile submarines USS Tecumseh SSBN 628 and USS Thomas Jefferson SSBN 618. He earned his D.P.M. at the California College of Podiatric Medicine in San Francisco in 1976.

Running and sports have been a large part of Zamzow's life, beginning in high school when he was captain of the track team. He is founder and president of the California Road Runners running club; vice chairman of The Athletics Congress (TAC), Pacific Association; advisor to the California Governor's Council on Wellness and Physical Fitness and a member of the Executive Board of the California Governor's Council on Wellness and Physical Fitness, San Jose chapter. He has instructed a marathon training class at De Anza College in Cupertino, California, and founded the California Road Runners 100-Mile Endurance Run. He has written many sports-related medical articles and is currently writing a book on

143

ultramarathoning. Zamzow's hobbies include flying (private pilot fourteen years), weightlifting and playing guitar. He directs many local races and has lectured extensively on sportsmedicine and podiatric surgery. Zamzow is listed in the 1982 edition of *Who's Who In The West*.

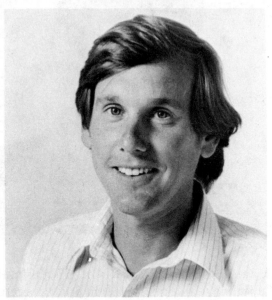

William P. Feigel, D.P.M.

William P. Feigel is a native of Philadelphia. He currently resides in San Jose, California, and has a private practice in nearby Mountain View. He is on staff at El Camino Hospital in Mountain View. Feigel served in the Vietnam war from 1967 to 1969. He attended the College of San Mateo and Stanford University, where he received a B.S. degree in biology. His D.P.M. was earned at the California College of Podiatric Medicine in San Francisco in 1978. Feigel also holds a B.S. degree in basic medical sciences. He completed surgical residency at Northlake Hospital in Chicago and returned to the West Coast in 1979 to set up private practice. His professional interests are sportsmedicine and podiatric surgery and he is board-eligible in the American Board of Podiatric Surgery. Feigel has written several sports-related medical articles for national publications and is writing a novel.

Recommended Reading

The following books, also available from Anderson World, can augment your exercise and fitness program. They are available from major bookstores or can be ordered directly from the publisher (1400 Stierlin Road, Mountain View, CA 94043).

RUNNER'S WORLD YOGA BOOK by Jean Couch with Nell Weaver. An easy-to-follow guide to using the principles of yoga for stretching, strengthening, and toning the body, and a good book to graduate to after you've outgrown some of the exercise routines in Runner's World Indoor Exercise Book. Spiral bound, $11.95.

TOTAL WOMAN'S FITNESS GUIDE by Gail Shierman, Ph.D., and Christine Haycock, M.D. A good guide to choosing a fitness program that fits your needs, your goals, and your lifestyle, with special attention to what happens to a woman's body during physical activity. Quality paperback, $4.95.

RUNNER'S WORLD INDOOR EXERCISE BOOK by Richard Benyo and Rhonda Provost. A simple-to-understand guide to fitness and the exercising body, and how it responds to beginning exercise programs. Programs are keyed to the beginner and oriented toward getting started comfortably indoors before moving into outdoor fitness training and outdoor sports. Spiral bound $11.95; Paperback $9.95.

GETTING YOUR EXECUTIVES FIT by Don T. Jacobs, Ph.D. The book that America's corporations have been waiting for. A book that, in one package, reviews all available facts on corporate fitness, while making the information accessible to everyone—from hourly worker to chairman of the board. Large-format paperback, $12.95.

THE FOOT BOOK by Harry F. Hlavac. A one-volume encyclopedia of the foot. Valuable reference guide containing technical information and practical advice. Hardback, $14.95.

RUNNER'S WORLD WEIGHT CONTROL BOOK by Michael Nash. A logical, realistic approach to losing weight and keeping it off forever that ignores the fad diets and gets right to the root of the problem: one's own image of self. Spiral bound, $11.95; paperback, $9.95.

DANCE AEROBICS by Maxine Polley. The rage that has swept the nation. Getting in shape and staying there through an ambitious program of enjoyable, fast-moving dance that builds aerobic fitness while toning muscles and doing away with unwanted weight. Quality paperback, $5.95

RUNNER'S WORLD MASSAGE BOOK by Ray Hosler. This is a book written by an inquiring journalist who looks at the new holistic massage. Over 140 photos take the reader stroke-by-stroke through a full body massage, as described and shown by two massage practitioners. The different massage techniques are experienced by the author, who gives his personal account of how he enjoyed them. The physiological effect of massage and how it can be used in sports is also detailed. Spiral bound $11.95, Paperback $9.95.

RUNNER'S WORLD STRENGTH TRAINING BOOK by Edwin Sobey. A complete program of strengthening without bulking is provided the reader interested in lifting weights. Photos illustrate the different and basic lifts, such as curls and the bench press, as well as the new Nautilus machines. The author also provides a complete stretching program that can be implemented with the weight workouts. Twenty-one sports-weight-training programs are listed, from running to archery, in this 186-page book. Spiral bound $11.95; paperback $9.95.

DR. SHEEHAN ON RUNNING by George A. Sheehan, M.D. This was the first of Dr. Sheehan's best-selling books on running. Reading Sheehan is a great way to spend a lazy afternoon. There is not only lively reading here, but the running doctor takes the reader through the basics of what makes the body tick, and how running makes it keep better time. Paperback, $4.95.

Everybody's Getting
Fit!

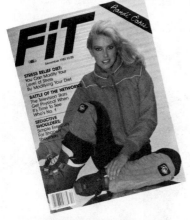
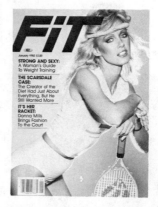

All over America millions of women are discovering that the key to self-esteem is feeling good and looking fit. And whether you're a business executive, a mother of five, a student or an athlete, *Fit* magazine is designed for *you*.

To help in your progress toward total fitness, *Fit* presents articles on the most revolutionary ideas on nutrition and diet; innovative exercise programs — including our new program of Sexercise — the most current information on health clubs, spas and vacation resorts; sound medical advice; career guidelines for successful women to follow; a look at the top athletic performers and trendsetters of our time; beauty, hair and skin consultations developed especially for fitness-conscious women; and the ever-changing world of international fashion.

Fit magazine has it all: provocative editorials written by the foremost professionals in their chosen fields; bold, compelling photography and graphics; and a style and energy that serve as a catalyst for *Fit* women everywhere.

So, come on and join the fitness explosion! *Fit* magazine wants you feeling strong, healthy and looking great . . . we'll be growing right along with you as your world broadens into the future. For only $14.95, you can receive the next 12 big, colorful issues of *Fit*.

Yes, I want to join everybody who's getting *Fit*. I have enclosed $14.95 for the next 12 big issues.

☐ Bill me

☐ Payment enclosed

☐ Charge my ☐ Visa ☐ MasterCard

\# _____ Exp. Date _____

Name _____

Address _____

City _____ State _____ Zip _____

Train With The Experts

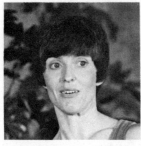

Jean Couch

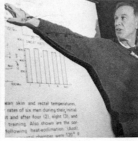

Dr. George Sheehan

Bill Dellinger

For 16 years, *Runner's World* has provided America's 25 million runners with the finest running publication possible.

As the world of running has evolved, so has *Runner's World.* It has grown from a single subscriber in 1966 to 1,248,000 readers every month.

Here's the reason why: *Runner's World* has consistently presented indispensable information and advice from the fitness experts of our times — the trainers and professionals who have mapped out the runner's road from the first step, on onward.

For example, *Runner's World* has printed the work of Dr. George Sheehan, nationally respected cardiologist, seasoned pro and author of numerous books and articles that offer medical knowledge and philosophical teachings.

Guidance from champions such as Tom Osler, long distance runner and author of *Ultramarathoning: The Next Challenge*. Mr. Osler's ground-breaking efforts continually provide fresh incentives for running enthusiasts everywhere.

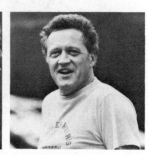

Discipline from leaders such as Jean Couch, whose words and instruction have opened the field of yoga to the running public.

And ardent support form coaches like University of Oregon great, Bill Dellinger, and Brooks Johnson, Stanford University's first-rate track-and-field leader.

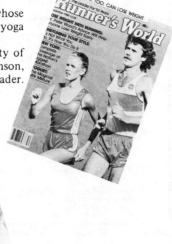

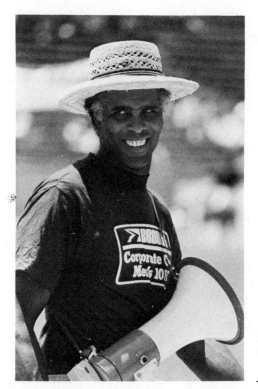

Brooks Johnson

All catalysts. All innovators. These concerned and committed professionals — and many others — have strived to build a bridge of communication to reach the running audience in this country and abroad. Together, they form a vital link to the future.

At *Runner's World,* we are proud to remain an integral part of this process. We welcome your continued support along the way to an increasingly energized, informed and trained "runner's world."